MANAGING A VETERINARY PRACTICE IN CANADA

Douglas C. Jack, BA, LLB

W.B. Saunders Canada
a division of
Harcourt Brace & Company, Canada
Toronto, Philadelphia, London, Sydney, Tokyo

W.B. Saunders Canada
a division of
Harcourt Brace & Company Canada, Ltd.
55 Horner Avenue
Toronto, Ontario M8Z 4X6

Managing a Veterinary Practice in Canada

ISBN 0-920513-11-5

Canadian Cataloguing in Publication Data

Jack, Douglas C.
Managing a veterinary practice in Canada

Includes index
ISBN 0-920513-11-5

1. Veterinary medicine - Practice - Canada
I. Title.

SF756.4.J33 1994   636.089'068   C94-930397-6

COVER PHOTO: James Burnett Photography Studios, Fergus, Ontario
DESIGN/DESKTOP PUBLISHING: Rick Eskins
EDITING: Kathleen Johnson
PRODUCTION: Francine Geraci

Printed in Canada at Webcom Limited
Last digit is print number: 9 8 7 6 5 4 3 2 1

CONTENTS

13   PROFESSIONAL ETHICS   141

APPENDIXES

TO DEBBIE

FOREWORD

The professional training of Canadian veterinarians is second to none; nonetheless, new graduates are often unprepared to deal with the legal and business aspects of managing a practice. We are not trained as lawyers, accountants, or business managers, but we require information from those related professions in order to carry on a successful practice. The prudent utilization of information found in this book will help to create a sound business environment, thereby promoting high-quality medicine, income enhancement, and higher levels of personal satisfaction.

Douglas Jack's important work on the legal aspects of veterinary practice management provides an indispensable guide for those wishing to establish or revive a practice. It is important to note that this work was prepared specifically for veterinarians by a highly qualified lawyer who understands the problems we face in business. His experience and dedication are revealed in the presentation of complex issues in a highly readable form.

The book sensitizes the reader to the key legal and business issues that may (and probably will) arise in the history of any practice. Anyone starting or buying a practice should read the book from cover to cover: all of the information is relevant. The material ranges from the problems of starting a practice to a discussion of the impact of family law, and always touches on the real issues of running a veterinary business.

Practice points are highlighted throughout the text, allowing for easy identification of important management principles. The extensive appendixes include a wide variety of legislative extracts and sample documents, which supplement the text on issues from partnership agreements to property division in the case of divorce. Now, for the first time, Canadian veterinarians have this material available in a concise and readable format.

This book is a fine demonstration of the way in which one profession can make a significant contribution to the more effective operation of another.

Donal B. McKeown, DVM

PREFACE

I wish I could say that my involvement in veterinary law was carefully planned and the result of a meticulous strategy. That is not the case. My development of this specialty was a pure accident of geography. My practice is located in Fergus, Ontario, which is very close to the Ontario Veterinary College at the University of Guelph. A few years ago I was invited by an accountant friend of mine to deliver some short lectures at OVC on employment and partnership law issues for senior veterinary students. I readily accepted the invitation — an invitation that led to the writing of this book.

In those earlier days I was honoured to meet Dr. Brent Matthew, who was then in charge of the course on professional affairs at OVC. Through my relationship with Dr. Matthew, who specializes in the business aspects of veterinary practice through his own consulting firm, I became aware of the profession's acute need for assistance in management. Much uncertainty prevailed among veterinary practitioners about partnership rights, employee relations, and disciplinary matters, and it was obvious that their practices were suffering financially because of their stress, worry, and fear of the unknown. It was important that those stresses be relieved.

From those initial lectures, other opportunities grew. Short articles in veterinary publications followed, as did speaking engagements for OVC continuing education modules, the first Canadian Conference of the Veterinary Hospital Managers Association, and the Ontario Veterinary Medical Association. The network of veterinarians, educators, and other consultants grew. In July 1993 Dr. Jim Wilson, a lawyer and veterinarian practising in Pennsylvania, invited me to attend the inaugural meeting of the American Veterinary Law Association. As the only Canadian lawyer in attendance, I was grateful to Jim for his kindness in including me in this group, which those veterinarians interested in management issues will hear much more about in the years to come.

My thanks for encouragement in this project are heartily extended to Marty Smart-Wilder, the executive director of the Ontario Veterinary Medical Association, and Dr. John Henry, the registrar of the College of Veterinarians of Ontario. One of my strongest mentors in this project has been Dr. Donal

McKeown, a client, fellow Rotarian, and friend. Don's inquiries throughout the writing of this book and his constant interest have been of more help to me than I can express.

My law partners deserve special mention. Weekly partnership meetings often included a report from me on how this area of our practice was developing. Thankfully, this specialty has grown faster than I or my partners would have imagined. Their indulgence in permitting me to use the services of office staff in the production of some of the elements of this text and in giving me the time to attend lectures and similar functions is greatly appreciated. My partner, Bob Grant, contributed much of the material in chapter 12 relating to family law in Ontario.

The first draft of the text was not completed when I received a call from Gerry Mungham, the acquisitions editor of W.B. Saunders Company. Gerry has been helpful in explaining the publication process and I have appreciated his candour throughout. I also wish to thank my editor, Kathleen Johnson, for her helpful and necessary suggestions, which have made the text more readable.

Finally, my thanks go out to my wife, Debbie, and my wonderful children, Martha, Emma, and Hannah. They have been subjected to my apparently endless thinking out loud and to countless hours of my sitting in front of a computer screen. I am grateful to them for much more than their patience and encouragement.

The purpose of this text is to highlight a number of legal issues that should assist the reader in managing a veterinary practice. It is not intended to be comprehensive or authoritative; rather, it has been written for the purpose of making the veterinarian and veterinary assistant more aware of the legal implications of some of the management decisions they will make. Legal advice is not provided here, and the reader is encouraged to seek professional assistance for specific legal problems.

As a matter of constitutional law, the provinces have exclusive jurisdiction on most issues involving veterinary practice; thus, a review of the legislation in each province has been undertaken. That being stated, I have erred on the side of citing laws and examples based on Ontario law, having regard to the recent amendments to the Ontario Veterinarians Act. Similarities and differences in other provincial legislation are pointed out. The case law cited is in no way exhaustive of the cases relating to veterinarians.

Robertson's Point, New Brunswick

July 1994

INTRODUCTION

In recent years, many professionals have come to recognize the importance of effective practice management and planning. With a volatile economy, more competition, more knowledgeable consumers, and rapid changes in technologies, veterinarians, like lawyers, accountants, engineers, physicians, and architects, must take active steps to ensure that their practices operate efficiently and effectively. Technical excellence is no longer the only criterion of a successful practice. The objective is not only to survive in practice, but to create sustainable profits.

The prudent veterinarian will have a sound knowledge of basic legal and business principles in order to effectively manage his or her practice. The conceptual benchmark to adopt is one of *certainty* — to know that by taking a specific course of action a given result is likely to occur. Adopting such a perspective lessens the anxiety that flows from having to accept a risk that, through proper planning, could have been easily avoided.

Every veterinarian possesses the professional expertise to carry on a veterinary practice. The granting of your long-awaited DVM shows that you have fulfilled the technical requirements to practice in the profession; however, the degree does not ensure your success in achieving good practice management. Veterinary schools in Canada and the United States have only begun to offer courses devoted to management issues as part of the curriculum. At least two provincial advocacy groups — in Ontario and Manitoba — have commissioned economic studies of the veterinary profession against which practitioners in those provinces might gauge the financial success of their practice.

While you should not expect to become an expert in veterinary law, it is necessary that you have an appreciation of essential legal principles and how they affect your day-to-day management decisions. Such an appreciation will give you a competitive advantage in your community and enable you to make business decisions with a view to avoiding problems that often have a substantial financial and emotional cost. Simply put, if you can identify a problem before it is elevated to a crisis, you will operate a more effective animal hospital.

In the most pragmatic sense, your goal is the operation of your practice to earn profit. No doubt you have other objectives in mind — satisfying your humanitarian and philanthropic sensibilities, working with animals, and ensuring their welfare. The fulfilment of those goals can be achieved only by the daily operation of a successful and profitable veterinary hospital.

Within the last few years various practice management special interest groups, small and large, formal and informal, have started to develop. This is clear evidence that veterinarians in Canada have recognized the importance of treating their professional practice as a business and a profit centre. The number of full-time practice administrators and managers has grown in recent years, and the official publications of the provincial veterinary associations contain regular columns on management issues. Many practitioners hire public relations firms to assist them in marketing their professional services to the public. While advertising is still restricted under provincial legislation, veterinarians throughout Canada are beginning to appreciate the advantages associated with educating the public with respect to the services available. Those who pay little attention to this aspect of their practice proceed at their peril.

In addition to good client relationships, the successful practitioner will enjoy a good relationship with the bank. The development of a business plan, for example, not only serves the internal needs of the practice, but is also available for review by the bank in connection with any application for credit. Knowing the types of loans and the collateral security normally requested by banks will assist you in negotiating the best arrangement for credit. Similarly, a basic knowledge of federal tax law and the operations of Revenue Canada will help you make better taxation-related business decisions. And, of course, effective client management is as important as the science necessary to perform veterinary medicine. Knowledgeable handling of client complaints and familiarity with the provincial disciplinary processes will lessen the cost and the stress associated with them.

While our discussion will be devoted mainly to the operation of your practice, it is important to deal with the maintenance of the wealth created from your active operations through effective personal and estate planning. Family law has a direct impact on the financial aspects of your practice and your relationship with your partners and associates. Through effective estate planning, your financial gains can be passed on to family and other beneficiaries upon your death.

My intention is to provide you with a discussion of key legal issues that will at some point require your attention in the successful operation of your clinic. The text is interspersed with a number of practice points to highlight some important facts and suggestions. To the extent that you can identify and react appropriately to legal issues, you will maintain an effective competitive edge and operate a more profitable clinic.

METHODS OF CARRYING ON PRACTICE

A veterinary practice may be structured as a sole proprietorship, as a partnership, as a co-ownership, or through the use of a corporation. Making the right decision about which form to use is important. The decision can have far-reaching implications for, among other things, your personal liability and taxation. The choice can be difficult to make, and will depend on a number of factors, all of which should be thoroughly analysed by you and your professional advisers.

In this portion of the text we will discuss the legal characteristics of each business entity, and examine its advantages and disadvantages with a view to determining whether your existing practice is being conducted in the most beneficial manner. A new practice will be subject to similar considerations.

SOLE PROPRIETORSHIP

By far, the simplest form of practice organization is that of a sole proprietorship. A sole proprietorship exists whenever an individual practitioner carries on practice on his or her own account.

LIABILITY

The sole practitioner owns the practice; he or she retains all the benefits of the practice and is subject to all its liabilities. The revenues and expenses of the practice belong to the owner, as does the equipment used in the clinic. The owner is personally responsible for carrying out the practice's contractual obligations — for instance, under a lease of the premises from which the clinic conducts its operations. All liabilities that arise out of the acts of the owner or his or her employees are the owner's sole responsibility; however, some of these obligations can be adequately limited by a policy of insurance or by engaging in a form of judgment proofing (discussed below). Unlike a corporation, a sole proprietorship is not a distinct legal entity. The practitioner is, for legal purposes, the only person who benefits from any success and suffers any failures.

As mentioned above, the sole proprietorship is the simplest way of carrying on a practice; there are few legal formalities other than the possible need to register a business name (as is the case in Ontario under the Business Names Act and the applicable provincial legislation requiring the name to be registered with the provincial registrar). In Manitoba, the Business Names Registration Act specifically excludes from registration all professions that are regulated under an act of the Manitoba legislature; accordingly, veterinarians in that province are not subject to the provincial business name registration requirement.

In addition, most provincial veterinary legislation sets out strict regulations concerning the type of practice carried on, from small-animal clinics to large-animal clinics or mobile clinics, which are discussed in chapter 4.

PRACTICE POINT

Because a sole proprietor has no way to limit personal liability, the prudent practitioner will make sure that adequate policies of insurance are available to cover the broadest number of claims, including professional negligence, occupiers' liability, business interruption, and all other foreseeable claims.

TAXATION

The income or loss from the practice in any year must be included in the practitioner's income or losses from other sources during the year. The aggregate result is taxed under the Income Tax Act (Canada) at the tax rates applicable to individuals. At present, those rates range from about 26 percent of net income to 46 percent of net income in most provinces.

PARTNERSHIP

A partnership is formed when two or more persons carry on business together with a view to obtaining a profit. Like sole proprietorships, the partnership does not exist as a distinct legal entity apart from the owners of the practice; that is, the individuals achieve all the benefits and are personally responsible for all the liabilities of the firm. In most provinces each partner must be a licensed veterinarian. The Ontario Veterinarians Act requires that each of the partners be a member of the College of Veterinarians of Ontario and be licensed to carry on a veterinary medicine practice.

LIABILITY

Veterinarians who wish to practice together will commonly use the partnership structure to pool assets and expertise and share the burdens of a veterinary practice.

There are two types of partnerships: general partnerships and limited partnerships. In a general partnership, the liability for the practice's debts and obligations extends to all of the partners personally. This type of partnership arrangement is widely used by veterinarians. Limited partnerships are not a common veterinary business structure: suffice it to say that a limited partner can limit his or her own exposure to liability.

In a partnership, each partner can speak on behalf of the entire partnership and all of the other partners; accordingly, the acts of one partner bind all the partners. Each partner in a veterinary practice is responsible for the debts and obligations of the firm. In other words, all of a partner's personal assets could be used to satisfy a judgment granted against a partnership. This is true even if a partner incurred the obligation without the other partners' knowledge or consent. While the partner who incurs the obligation may have a duty to account to the remaining partners for his or her actions, a third party can rely, in most cases, upon the ability of one partner to contract on behalf of the whole firm.

The legal implications of partnerships and methods of more effectively managing your clinic through a partnership are discussed further in chapter 6.

PRACTICE POINT

Most veterinarians working together are involved in a form of partnership; however, many have failed to document the relationship properly. Many partnerships are carried on without any formal agreements. It is dangerous to operate in this manner, particularly with respect to the individual estate plans of the partners and the continuity of ownership of the practice. You have invested a great deal in your practice, both financially and emotionally; you should take active steps to preserve that investment.

TAXATION

Taxation of a partnership is somewhat different from taxation of a sole proprietorship in that the income and losses of the practice are determined at the partnership level. Expenses are deducted from the clinic's gross income to determine the net taxable income. That income is then divided among the partners in proportion to their partnership interests. Each partner then includes that income with all other sources of income to determine his or her net taxable income for the year. The individual partner is taxed at the applicable marginal rate of tax which, as mentioned earlier, varies from province to province.

CO-OWNERSHIP

In some cases veterinarians may want to carry on a practice in the same clinic, but not as partners. In this arrangement, each contributes to payment of the clinic's overhead expense — receptionist, technicians, groomers, office equipment, and professional equipment. In contrast to partnerships, the participants are not agents for one another and do not share in one another's liabilities. These co-ownership relationships are commonly referred to as space-sharing arrangements.

Great care must be taken in drafting a space-sharing agreement or contract to ensure that the relationship does not become a partnership. Effectively, each practitioner receives income from his or her own services and contributes to the expenses associated with the common premises.

CORPORATION

As previously mentioned, veterinarians are currently prohibited from incorporating their professional practices in some provinces; in others, they are permitted to incorporate, but under strict limitations. For tax purposes and for reasons of liability, some practitioners choose to incorporate a form of holding corporation, which owns the assets of the practice and leases them to the sole practitioner or partnership. In essence, the practitioner separates the professional activities of veterinary medicine from the business activity and ownership of the assets used in the practice.

LIABILITY

Unlike the other business structures discussed, a corporation is a separate legal entity. The corporation may own property, sell it, commence legal proceedings, and sue and be sued. The shareholders own the corporation through their shares. Many veterinarians arrange for the ownership of shares by their spouses. The shareholders do not own the practice or the property that belongs to the corporation; rather, they own the entity that owns the assets.

In order to obtain shares in the corporation, the shareholders may pay money for them or may provide services or property of value to the corporation. The shareholders' liability for the activities of the corporation is limited to the extent of the value of their shares in the corporation. The corporation's distinctiveness means that any lawsuit must be brought against the entity and not the shareholders that own the corporation. The creditors of the corporation can demand to be repaid from the assets of the corporation, but they cannot demand that the debt be repaid by the shareholders themselves. In most cases the shareholders will purchase shares that have nominal value. In this fashion the shareholder who in his or her personal activity may be exposed to professional liabilities will not have much at stake, in that he or she has made little investment. This limited liability can be lost if the shareholder signs a form of personal guarantee for the debts of the corporation. Most banks and other institutional lenders require such a guarantee when granting loans.

In a veterinary holding company, the veterinarian uses the equipment and other assets owned by the corporation and pays a user fee. To the extent that the user fee is paid to a corporation owned by the veterinarian and his or her spouse, income is generated in the holding corporation for later distribution to the shareholders. The veterinarian's professional fees fall into his or her net income calculation, while the user fee is paid to the corporation and, perhaps, paid out to the veterinarian's spouse.

In New Brunswick, incorporation of a veterinary practice is specifically permitted subject to certain rules in the provincial Veterinarians Act. Part IV of the New Brunswick legislation provides that such a professional corporation is not entitled to vote at any meeting of the New Brunswick Veterinary Medical Association; however, all of the legislated rules in the act and its bylaws apply to individual members and to professional corporations. The articles of incorporation cannot prevent the corporation from engaging in every "phase and aspect of rendering the same veterinary services to the public that a veterinarian is authorized to render," and an incorporated practice must have all the capacity of a natural person as may be incidental to the providing of veterinary services. These latter traits would include the ability to lease or acquire property, to enter into contracts, to enter into a partnership, and to purchase assets of another individual or corporation rendering similar services.

The main restriction in the New Brunswick statute is contained in section 21, which states that the legal and beneficial ownership of all the issued shares in the professional corporation shall be vested in one or more members of the professional association, and the attributes of the shares must include provisions that permit members to elect all the directors of the corporation. Further, the practice of veterinary medicine on behalf of such a veterinary corporation must be carried on by veterinarians or persons who are otherwise qualified according to the New Brunswick legislation.

In the event that any conditions contained in the New Brunswick act are unfulfilled or upon the death of an individual member of the association who owns shares in the corporation, the removal from the register of the member, or the suspension or revocation of any licence held by the individual member, the corporation has 180 days in which to correct the problem or fulfil the conditions, failing which the registrar of the association must revoke the licence of the corporation.

As previously indicated, one of the significant legal advantages to incorporation is the ability to insulate oneself from liability. The New Brunswick act, for the most part, removes that ability in sections 22 and

23 of the provincial Veterinarians Act. By virtue of section 22, the relationship of a member, whether as a shareholder, director, officer, or employee of a professional corporation, is not affected by or diminished from the application of the act, bylaws, or rules. Section 23 states that nothing in the legislation relating to professional corporations "affects, modifies or limits any ethical obligation of a veterinarian."

The rules relating to incorporation in New Brunswick are further detailed in bylaw 15 of the New Brunswick Veterinary Medical Association. The registrar is required to maintain a register of the name, registration number, address, and any other particulars of the corporation. Any registration made by the corporation under the New Brunswick Business Corporations Act or the Partnerships and Business Names Registration Act must also be made to the registrar. A specific form of information return must be made to the registrar by December 1 of each year. Bylaw 15.04 requires each corporation to appoint a member of the association as its representative, to whom all communications may be sent.

In Prince Edward Island, veterinarians are expressly permitted to incorporate their practices by section 6.1 of the Veterinary Profession Act. As is the case in New Brunswick, a number of restrictions are set out in the act: for instance, no corporation may charge a fee for the services of a person licensed to practise in that province unless the shares of the corporation are wholly owned by a person licensed to practise or by the spouse of such a person. As well, in the event that shares of the corporation are to be transferred to someone not licensed to practise veterinary medicine (except a bank as security for a loan), the council or executive of the PEI Veterinary Medical Association must be notified of the proposed transfer and must approve the transfer prior to its being effected.

Nova Scotia permits the incorporation of a veterinary practice, provided that the individual who conducts the practice is licensed to practise clinical veterinary medicine. As is the case in Prince Edward Island, no fees for veterinary services can be charged by a corporate practice unless all the issued shares of the corporation are beneficially owned by one or more persons who hold a licence to practise. As well, any transfers of shares must be approved by the council of the Nova Scotia Veterinary Medical Association. One interesting aspect of the Nova Scotia rules of share ownership is that shares owned by a spouse of a licensed veterinarian are deemed to be owned by the veterinarian. Thus, income splitting can be achieved between spouses without violating the provincial legislation.

TAXATION

Since the corporation is a distinct legal entity, it is taxed very differently from the individuals who own it. A corporation's net income is subject to tax each year, and any after-tax income can be distributed to the shareholders by way of a dividend on the shares. Corporations, unlike individuals, are subject to a flat rate of tax, which in Ontario is almost 50 percent of the net corporate income; however, some corporations carrying on small business are entitled to various deductions, which effectively reduce the rate of tax paid. This is discussed in more detail in chapter 8.

CHOOSING THE BEST METHOD

All veterinary practices must be carried on in one of the business structures referred to above. The prudent practitioner will give thoughtful consideration to a number of factors either before initiating a new practice or in re-evaluating his or her existing arrangements. A number of legal implications discussed throughout this text will flow directly from the business entity you select, from potential personal exposure to liability for the wrongful dismissal of an employee to developing an appropriate estate plan.

PERSONAL LIABILITY

The practice of veterinary medicine exposes the practitioner to some risks. Only the corporate structure limits your personal liability. Sole practitioners and partners in veterinary practice remain personally liable for the debts and obligations of the practice. You should consider taking some steps to limit that personal risk through the transfer of assets into the name of a spouse or other person when you commence your practice or as the assets are acquired. This judgment-proofing technique must be used before a liability arises in order to avoid a court finding that the assets were fraudulently transferred. No transfer can be effective if it was implemented solely for the purpose of defeating the claims of creditors. In provinces where incorporation is permitted, the practitioner's personal assets are protected through the very existence of a separate and distinct corporate entity; however, as further protection the divestiture of personal assets may be a good planning technique.

Adequate policies of professional liability insurance should be obtained to cover negligence claims, especially for large-animal practices, for which the amount claimed in any lawsuit could be quite high.

PRACTICE POINT

For the veterinarian who is starting out, it is imperative that thoughtful consideration be given to the legal entity used to conduct the practice. This is the first step in effective practice management. The success of your practice depends largely on knowing the implications of the business structure you have selected.

NUMBER OF PARTICIPANTS

It is clear that only a single owner can conduct a veterinary practice as a sole practitioner, and that at least two persons are required to carry on a partnership. A corporation may be established by one or more shareholders, subject to provincial securities laws, which often limit the number of shareholders necessary to maintain private corporation status.

LEGAL RESTRICTIONS

Regulatory authorities will have an impact on the business structure you select. Because veterinarians in some provinces are prohibited by law from incorporating the professional aspects of their practice, corporations may be used only as holding corporations and not for the delivery of professional veterinary services.

COSTS

The relative legal and accounting costs of starting or continuing a practice in any form often determine the method chosen. Generally, it is significantly less expensive to establish a sole proprietorship, which, apart from any mandatory name registrations, has few costs associated with it. For instance, the government fee for a name filing in Ontario at present is $60. The government fees for incorporation are significantly higher — $250 in Saskatchewan and $260 in Prince Edward Island. In addition, you should anticipate legal costs of up to $1,000 plus some accounting fees. The costs of establishing a partnership are minimal, except for the legal costs of drafting a comprehensive partnership agreement, which could be as high as $750 to $1,000.

Each method also carries some administrative costs in terms of accounting and other professional fees; however, those fees should not vary dramatically, regardless of the method selected. Corporations are required to have financial statements prepared by an accountant each year for presentation to the shareholders; however, most partnerships will want the benefit of these accounting statements as well.

STARTING A PRACTICE

The establishment or continuation of a veterinary practice is subject to a number of important considerations. The launching of a new practice can be an exciting venture, and many issues that arise in the special circumstances of your practice must be addressed. The acquisition of a practice is addressed in detail in chapter 3. What follows is a general discussion of some of the details to be considered.

COMMERCIAL LEASES

One legal document that significantly affects your practice is the lease of your premises. Many veterinarians consider the lease to be a "boilerplate" or "off-the-shelf" document. Such a notion is wrong, and can lead you to enter into a form of lease that can cause problems in your practice.

The location of a practice is key to its success, particularly when a practitioner is just starting out. The term, or length, of the lease should be tailored to the relative desirability of the premises: if the premises are in a highly visible, highly populated area, you will want to attempt to secure a long-term lease. If the premises are merely satisfactory, and "will do" until a better location is found, the term should be shortened. You should ascertain the terms for renewal of the lease at its expiry, and the costs associated with the renewal.

The typical form of rental arrangement in a commercial lease consists of the payment of a basic rent, together with the payment of additional rent relating to a contribution to the expenses of the landlord for the operation of the premises. Additional rent can include contributions to property taxes, insurance, maintenance, heating and air-conditioning, and snow removal. This type of lease is usually referred to as a "net, net lease": the basic rent received by the landlord is "net" of the landlord's expenses in operating the building.

The use of the premises is often restricted in the lease. Obviously, the use must include the operation of a veterinary practice; however, you should also determine whether the retail or wholesale sale of pet or animal products or boarding services should be included. In addition, you should be aware of "exclusivity clauses" to be appended so as to limit competition in the same building from other veterinary practices or ancillary services.

Unlike residential leases, a commercial lease is usually assignable to a third party only with the written consent of the landlord. The consent may be arbitrarily withheld; accordingly, care must be taken to ensure that the lease may be assigned or a sublease entered into.

A typical form of commercial lease is found in appendix A.

PRACTICE POINT

If you are leasing your premises, ensure that the term of the lease coincides with your business plan; in other words, if your business plan contemplates the attainment of certain objectives within five years, you should make sure that the plan will not be prejudicially affected by a sudden unanticipated relocation of your practice.

EQUIPMENT LEASES

The cost of specialized veterinary equipment can often be prohibitive to a new veterinarian. Many vendors will permit the veterinarian to lease the equipment for a period of time with or without an option to acquire it outright. In addition, a number of leasing firms offer leasing contracts in the event that the vendor itself does not. The rentals paid under an equipment lease are tax-deductible as a properly incurred expense of the practice.

MUNICIPAL ZONING

Before signing a property lease or purchasing a building or land upon which to build a clinic, it is vitally important to make sure that the location complies with the municipal zoning bylaw relating to the types of activities that can be carried on. For veterinary offices in residential neigh-bourhoods, care should be taken to ensure that the professional practice falls within the type of "home occupations" that may be lawfully carried on.

Many municipalities also regulate the number of parking spaces that must be made available to clients.

A breach of the zoning bylaws could result in a prosecution under the bylaw and an order to cease activities in breach of the rules.

PRACTICE POINT

When you are selecting a location for a veterinary practice, one of your first stops should be your local municipal offices. Try to speak with the zoning inspectors or the chief building official. These municipal em-ployees can be an invaluable source of information, and can help you to avoid many zoning pitfalls.

SHARING SPACE

As discussed in chapter 1, many new practitioners prefer to enter into a space-sharing arrangement, in which each party pays a share of the ex-penses of the premises. Such an arrangement must be carefully documented so as to ensure fairness and certainty.

GOODS AND SERVICES TAX

Before starting practice, a veterinarian must apply for and obtain a regis-tration number for the federal goods and services tax (GST), which must be charged on fees for professional activities and product sales.

GST must be remitted quarterly to Revenue Canada. The amount of tax to be remitted is equal to the amount of tax charged to clients, whether or not the account has been paid, less the amount of any GST paid by the prac-tice. This last amount is referred to as "input tax credits." In effect, you obtain a credit for any GST you have paid for supplies, rent, or other office expenses; that amount is offset against the amount of GST charged to clients.

MUNICIPAL LICENCES

You should check with the clerk or administrator of your municipality to determine whether a specific municipal licence must be obtained in order to carry on practice.

PROVINCIAL SALES TAX

A veterinary practice will require a vendor's permit or a retail sales tax permit if animal or pet products, including pet foods, are offered for sale. Various penalties are imposed for the failure to collect and remit retail sales tax.

CREDITOR PLANNING

The prudent veterinarian will take appropriate steps to ensure that his or her personal assets are not available to be seized or otherwise affected by the liabilities of the practice. Many professionals, in addition to obtaining negligence insurance, will take the precautionary step of transferring assets to spouses for the purpose of creditor-proofing those assets. This type of planning must be implemented before a liability arises; otherwise, such a transfer may be set aside as fraudulent.

SELECTING PROFESSIONAL ADVISERS

Many business decisions require the advice and expertise of other professionals, particularly lawyers and accountants. One of the best ways to find your advisers is through referrals from others. Approaching a trusted colleague to provide you with a recommendation is, in most cases, an excellent means of selecting someone who will have a significant impact on the success of your practice. Alternatively, you may want to use the lawyer referral services provided by the provincial law associations. For instance, the referral service maintained by the Law Society of Upper Canada contains a database of Ontario lawyers who provide specialized services in different areas of law. You may use the service free of charge: when you identify the area of law in which you need assistance, the service will give you the name of a lawyer in your geographic area who practises in the field. You are then provided with a one-half-hour free consultation with the lawyer to whom you were referred, so that you can decide whether you wish to engage him or her to act on your behalf.

Finally, a perusal of the local classified telephone directory will provide many names of accountants and lawyers; be sure to inquire whether the particular adviser you contact has experience and expertise in the matters in which you need assistance.

More important than the actual finding of an adviser is your ultimate selection of the person with whom you will be working in the course of your business activities. Above all, you must feel comfortable with the advice that is provided to you, and you must be able to work cooperatively with your advisers if the relationship is to last. Be sure to inquire about the costs that you are likely to incur on any particular matter; your adviser should show no reluctance to inform you fully in that regard.

Your legal and financial advisers are more than mere "hired guns" engaged to deal with specific matters as they arise. You will want to develop a relationship with them so that you can consult with them on a broad range of issues, knowing that you will receive thoughtful advice. Your professional advisers will have significant input in some of the decisions you make in your practice, and you must feel comfortable not only with the quality of the advice given but with your continuing relationship.

PURCHASE AND SALE OF A PRACTICE

In all businesses, including your veterinary practice, three clear parts of the business cycle emerge: acquisition, operation, and disposition. The successful practitioner recognizes which phase he or she is in at any given time, and constantly makes plans for the next phase.

In this chapter we will look at two types of transactions involving the acquisition or disposition of a practice: either the purchase of the assets that make up the practice, or the acquisition of the shares of a corporation that owns the assets. As well, we will investigate various means of initiating internal transfers of interests between shareholders or partners. The discussion will highlight the fact that the vendor and purchaser often have divergent interests, a situation that calls for skillful negotiation tactics.

In these materials I have adopted the purchaser's perspective; however, the effects of the agreement on the vendor in certain areas are addressed.

ASSET TRANSACTIONS

The typical method of acquiring a veterinary practice is through the purchase of the assets of an existing clinic from a veterinary practitioner or partnership. This is known as the "purchase of assets as a going concern." The new owners are able to commence operations immediately, as all of the necessary assets are available after the closing of the deal.

The purchaser acquires the practice by purchasing all or some of the assets that make up the existing enterprise, including drugs, equipment, goodwill, clinic name, accounts receivable, land and buildings, and client lists.

The primary advantage of purchasing assets from a vendor who is a sole practitioner, a veterinary partnership, or a corporation is the purchaser's ability to select only those assets he or she desires and to avoid the liabilities of the vendor. The dramatic difference between the purchase of assets and the purchase of shares is that with the latter tactic the buyer acquires both the benefits and liabilities of the corporation that has issued the shares. Some of the liabilities will be unknown, such as those revealed on a tax audit of the prior year's corporate taxes.

Probably the most useful way of looking at the acquisition of assets is to review the common provisions contained in an asset purchase agreement. AppendixB is a typical form of asset purchase agreement, which sets out the concerns to which a purchaser should direct his or her mind in the negotiation process. Each of those areas is commented upon briefly below.

NEGOTIATION ISSUES

Apart from the significant tax considerations that accompany the negotiation of any agreement to purchase the assets of a veterinary practice, other important legal and financial matters must be discussed.

Identity of Assets

It is imperative that a detailed list of all assets being purchased be included in the agreement of purchase and sale. To this end, it is often convenient to annex a schedule to the agreement, setting out all those assets that are included, complete with information such as serial numbers and quantity. Equipment such as radiographs or autoclaves will be set out in such a list.

Inventory

Often the value to be ascribed to an inventory of drugs or other treatment aids is a matter of opinion. The agreement should indicate a method of taking inventory before closing, together with a manner in which the value attached to the items can be objectively determined. Typically, the inventory will be valued at the lower of the vendor's cost or its fair market value. As well, the purchaser should beware the purchase of any outdated or obsolete inventory. For instance, certain drugs will carry near-term expiry dates which have little or no value.

Clinic Name

One of the most important assets of a practice is the clinic name. Special consideration must be given to the inclusion of a provision that requires the vendor to cease using the name. Remember that the provincial regulatory bodies must be advised of the new use of the clinic name, and the practice must be registered under that name with the profession's governing body.

Land and Buildings

If the purchase is to include the land and buildings from which the clinic operates, special provisions must be included so that inspections and title searches can be completed and reported upon before the closing date. For instance, when you acquire the lands it must be determined that there are no mortgages or other liens registered against the title to the property and that there are no property tax arrears.

Lease

In the event that the vendor is not the owner of the lands and premises from which the veterinary practice is carried on, the purchaser must obtain a warranty from the vendor that a valid lease is in effect, together with a covenant from the vendor that he or she will obtain the consent of the landlord to an assignment of the lease. The purchaser should always obtain a copy of the lease before entering the agreement of purchase and sale so as to ensure that the provisions are satisfactory, and in particular that the term of the lease is of sufficient length to continue the practice.

Telephone Number

In some cases the telephone number used by the vendor is a significant asset because it is well known to clients and to the public at large. The agreement between a vendor and purchaser should contain a provision wherein the vendor grants the use of the telephone number to the purchaser and directs the telephone authorities to permit such a transfer. Details of any directory advertising should be provided, including the cost and layout of same.

Purchase Price

The determination of the purchase price of the assets is strictly a matter of negotiation between a willing vendor and a willing purchaser. The agreement should specify whether or not the value of inventory is included or excluded from the purchase price. A deposit from the purchaser is usually provided as an indication of goodwill, and will be forfeited if the transaction is aborted as a result of the purchaser's failure to honour the contract.

For tax purposes, it is important to provide for an allocation of the purchase price among the various assets being acquired. All too often transactions run into difficulty when the vendor and purchaser enter into an agreement and later cannot agree on an appropriate allocation. Many important tax issues should be reviewed at the time the agreement is prepared; this topic is discussed in more detail below.

Accounts Receivable

If accounts receivable are to be purchased, there should be a representation by the vendor that they are collectable. The purchaser should have some right of recourse against the vendor for those that prove not to be. Most practices, except for some large-animal practices, will not have significant accounts receivable.

PRACTICE POINT

In most acquisitions of veterinary practices, assets rather than shares will be purchased. If a holding corporation is used in the practice to be transferred, the vendor may prefer to sell shares so as to maximize the tax benefits available to him or her. Purchasers of shares of a holding corporation also acquire the disclosed and undisclosed liabilities of the corporation. A properly drafted agreement of purchase and sale is vital in a share transaction.

EMPLOYMENT MATTERS

The labour costs inherent in the purchase are an important factor to be considered in your negotiations. If the number of employees is to be reduced by the purchaser, the cost of the reduction and who shall bear it must be determined. Provincial employment standards legislation dictates that on the sale of substantially all of the assets of a business, where the employment relationships are continued the employees are deemed to have been employed in the new practice retrospectively to the date of first employment by the vendor. This can have a major impact in the event of the subsequent dismissal of a continuing employee (as discussed in chapter 5).

PRACTICE POINT

Purchasers of a practice must pay special attention to the continued employment of the vendor's employees. Recent decisions by the Employment Standards Branch of the Ontario Ministry of Labour have indicated that, notwithstanding that the vendor has paid severance claims, the purchaser may, upon termination of the assumed employee, be required to pay a severance claim dating back to the date of first employment with the vendor.

RETAIL SALES TAX

Section 4 of the Ontario Retail Sales Tax Act provides that the purchaser becomes liable for retail sales tax payable by the vendor in the event that a clearance from the Retail Sales Tax Branch of the Ontario Ministry of Revenue is not obtained. A clearance certificate must be provided to the purchaser by the vendor on or before the closing date. This will generally affect practices where the sales of pet food or accessories take place. Similarly, sales tax statutes of those provinces where sales tax is applicable provide that the purchaser must ensure that any applicable tax has been remitted by the vendor.

NON-COMPETITION COVENANTS

A purchaser would be very disheartened to find the vendor opening a new clinic across the street the day after closing. Any benefit of goodwill that was paid for by the purchaser would surely be lost. Therefore, it is usual to obtain from the vendor a covenant not to compete in a similar business in a specific area for a period of time which, in order to be enforceable, must be reasonable. Generally, such covenants are not enforceable unless they are limited in time and restricted to a geographic location. A broad covenant not to compete at all would not be lawful.

PRACTICE POINT

The non-competition covenant must be very carefully drafted, because such terms are generally not enforceable unless they are reasonable. Much of the goodwill of a practice lies in the personalities of the veterinarians and the development of client relationships. The purchaser of a practice will be severely affected if the vendor reopens a clinic in a short distance of the acquired practice.

SHARE TRANSACTIONS

As mentioned in chapter 1, in some provinces veterinarians are not permitted to incorporate their professional practice; however, some practitioners transfer their assets to a holding corporation and then pay a user fee or a lease payment for the use thereof. In provinces such as New Brunswick and Nova Scotia, where incorporation is allowed under certain guidelines, practitioners have the additional advantage of disposing of their practices by selling the shares. This separates the ownership of the assets from the actual practice of veterinary medicine and the connected risks of liability. From chapter 1, we know that the shareholders represent the owners of all the assets and liabilities of a corporation; thus, the second method of acquiring a practice is through the purchase of shares from the shareholders or from a corporation which owns all the assets and liabilities of the practice.

Generally, the shareholders of a veterinary corporation will want to sell the shares of the corporation because the disposition of shares normally gives rise to a capital gain, which attracts beneficial tax treatment. The gain is taxed at a low rate, and a lifetime capital gains exemption was available for up to $100,000 (and in some cases $500,000, depending on the nature of the corporation). This exemption has been abolished in the federal budget of February 1994; assuming that the budget is adopted, the taxpayer has until the end of the 1994 tax year to elect to treat gains as exempt up to the $100,000 limit. The specific exemptions for agricultural business and small corporations remain intact.

That method is not always desirable to the purchaser. Since the purchaser is acquiring a corporation, he or she is also obtaining all the liabilities of the corporation. In other words, the purchaser gets the good with the bad. To combat the risk of these liabilities, the purchaser generally obtains a number of warranties from the vendor that all the corporation's liabilities have been disclosed and that the financial statements accurately reflect the financial condition of the corporation. The purchaser must be aware of liabilities for income taxes, sales taxes, and pending court proceedings. If the vendor gives such a warranty and it later proves to be untrue, the purchaser has a legal right to pursue compensation from the vendor for breach of warranty. As further protection, the purchaser could seek a form of indemnity from the vendor whereby the vendor promises to pay to the purchaser any monies the purchaser has had to pay as a result of an untrue warranty.

In addition, special provisions should be included in the agreement to ensure that the corporate records have been maintained and are up to date and that the corporation has complied with all federal, provincial, and municipal laws up to the closing date. Usually this is provided by way of an opinion letter from the solicitors of the vendor corporation confirming that the requirements have been satisfied.

PRACTICE POINT

Under some provincial legislation it is necessary to file a notice of changes in the directors, officers, and registered office of a corporation to the ministry in charge of incorporations. You should ensure that those filings are attended to if you purchase the shares of a veterinary corporation.

Finally, the agreement will provide for the resignation of the officers and directors of the corporation and the transfer of the shares that are the subject matter of the transaction. The corporate records must be amended to reflect the new owners' positions as officers and directors of the corporation, and new share certificates must be issued to the purchasers.

In the event that the purchase price is payable in part at the closing date and in part at some later time, the vendor must consider the type of collateral security that is required to secure any unpaid portion of the purchase price. The most obvious assets on which to take security are the assets of the corporation whose shares are being acquired. As well, a pledge of the shares that are the subject matter of the transaction may be provided to the vendor.

TAX CONSIDERATIONS: ASSET TRANSACTIONS

One of the issues deserving of careful negotiation with respect to the acquisition of a practice is whether or not a purchaser will buy assets or, in the case of a corporate vendor, the shares of the vendor. Obviously, the latter will be possible only if the vendor carries on practice with the assistance of a holding corporation that owns the assets of the practice. Generally speaking, the vendor will want to sell the shares of the corporation because the gain he or she will realize will be a capital gain and either exempt from income tax or effectively taxed at lower rates. The purchaser will want to buy assets, so that he or she will not be subject to any undisclosed liabilities and will have the opportunity to increase the capital cost of the assets to obtain tax deductions for depreciation as the practice continues.

Special tax considerations in an asset transaction will include the following.

DEPRECIABLE PROPERTY

Many of the assets used in a practice, including veterinary equipment, are depreciable property insofar as they are eligible for the capital cost allowance (CCA). The CCA is a significant factor in negotiating the allocation of the purchase price of depreciable property. The rate of depreciation is based on a fixed percentage established under the income tax legislation, and varies depending on the nature of the equipment; for instance, a motor vehicle will depreciate at a different rate from computer equipment or computer software used in the practice.

Throughout the life of the practice the vendor has taken the CCA, which gives rise in each fiscal year to an undepreciated capital cost value of a particular asset at a given time. To the extent that the agreement provides for an allocation of the purchase price of that asset in excess of the undepreciated capital cost, the vendor will suffer recapture. Recapture is a method by which the excess amount is added to your income for tax purposes, resulting in an increase in the amount of tax payable. Nevertheless, the purchaser will want to set the allocation price as high as possible, since that figure forms the adjusted cost base from which depreciation or CCA deductions will accrue to him or her. Since depreciation is calculated as a fixed percentage of the capital cost of the asset, the greater the value assigned to it, the greater the amount of the depreciation deduction.

LAND

The regulations to the Income Tax Act set out various rates at which the CCA may be taken on various types of depreciable property. Land cannot be depreciated for tax purposes, and any profit made on the sale of the land will be considered a capital gain. Thus, it is important to arrive at a negotiated allocation figure for land, because any portion of the sale price in excess of the original cost will result in a capital gain to the vendor, which will be taxed at effectively lower rates, while the purchaser will receive little or no benefit from a high allocation, since it cannot be depreciated and a large allocation reduces the purchaser's chance to obtain any significant capital gain upon resale.

PRACTICE POINT

The allocation of the practice's purchase price should be carefully reviewed by your accounting and tax advisers. An improper allocation can have grave consequences in terms of recapture for the vendor.

GOODWILL

Goodwill is an asset of the vendor, and is defined as the vendor's ability to generate income that has value over and above the worth of the practice assets as defined by their ability to generate income. Goodwill may be a reflection of the vendor's personality, the location of the business, or the clinic's reputation.

Under the Income Tax Act, goodwill falls into the category of eligible capital property. Three-quarters the goodwill amount is called the eligible capital amount. This amount is entitled to be depreciated at the rate of 7 percent per year. When the vendor sells goodwill, the amount by which the goodwill allocation exceeds the balance remaining in the vendor's eligible capital account is added into the vendor's income (similar to recapture). Therefore, it is important that the parties address this allocation issue.

TAX CONSIDERATIONS: SHARE TRANSACTIONS

In addition to the initial tax issues negotiated between the purchaser and the vendor with respect to the relative merits of purchasing assets or purchasing shares (the latter of which, you will recall, gives rise to a capital gain for the vendor), there are a number of other tax issues to be dealt with in the share transaction.

PRIOR YEARS' TAXES

There may be tax liability in dispute from prior years. Revenue Canada has three years in which to reassess prior years' taxes and longer if the reassessment results in a determination that fraud or misrepresentation has occurred. The purchaser may take some comfort if prior years have been audited by Revenue Canada and there has been no reassessment and no items are still outstanding for those years, as there is little likelihood of a further tax assessment. It is very important that the purchaser assess the degree of exposure for these potential liabilities.

PRACTICE POINT

One method of protecting yourself from an untrue vendor's warranty with respect to the payment of taxes is to obtain a form of indemnity that is binding on the vendor personally. Remember that the indemnity is only as valuable as the vendor's financial ability to pay any claim you might have against the vendor for breach of a warranty.

CURRENT AND FUTURE YEARS' TAXES

The purchaser should determine if tax instalments and source deductions for employees are up to date. A complete disclosure of the tax status of the corporation should be sought by the purchaser, as those liabilities, if any, will continue to exist after the transaction is completed.

OTHER TAX MATTERS

The scope of this work makes it difficult to discuss all of the far-reaching tax implications of a share purchase agreement; accordingly, both the purchaser and the vendor are well advised to discuss the entire transaction in detail with their respective tax advisers before entering into the agreement of purchase and sale.

INTERNAL TRANSFERS

In the event that one carries on business with other persons, either in a partnership or through a corporation, one of the matters that should be addressed is the manner in which the internal transfers — that is, the transfer of interests between existing owners, whether they are partners or shareholders of the ownership entity — are to be implemented.

To this end, it is very important that a partnership or shareholder agreement be entered into among all the principals of the practice. Among other things, the agreement may set out the employment functions, remuneration, benefits, accounting requirements, and other matters relating to the ongoing affairs of the business. More important, the agreement may also reflect the principals' interests upon termination of the relationship. There are a number of common provisions in partnership and shareholder agreements regarding the internal transfer of practice interests among partners or shareholders.

RIGHT OF FIRST REFUSAL

At the time of commencing a practice, the principals normally rely on the credibility and integrity of the various persons involved. Therefore, it is important for a clinic to maintain control over the continuity of ownership of the practice. In the event that one person wishes to leave the practice, it is a good idea to provide for a right of first refusal. Such a provision gives the remaining owners of the practice an option to acquire the departing individual's interest in the practice before an unknown third party becomes involved.

By this mechanism, the remaining parties are offered some protection against taking into the practice persons who, for personal or commercial reasons, are not conducive to a good business relationship. Such a provision does not unduly hinder the departing individual's rights to deal with his interests in the business.

BUY-SELL PROVISIONS

Another common means of effecting an internal transfer of interests in a veterinary practice is through a mandatory sale provision, commonly referred to as a buy-sell provision. A typical provision is reproduced in the partnership agreement in appendix C. In that example (a two-person partnership), a partner has the right to set a price for his or her partnership interest, while the other partner has the option of buying that interest for that price or selling his or her interest at that price. This is a reasonable and fair means of dealing the partnership interests, because the offeror-partner will be forced to choose a reasonable price, not knowing whether or not he or she will be receiving or paying cash. A usual precondition to the use of this type of clause is that the partners be of relatively equal financial strength.

The alternative to providing for the internal transfer of interests, especially if one party's expectations have not been realized, is either dissolution of the practice or litigation. Therefore, the buy-sell provision, coupled with a mechanism for valuing the interest of the principals, is an expeditious, enforceable, and less expensive means of dealing with the problem.

We have looked at two of the three time periods in the business cycle: acquisition and disposition. The successful purchase or sale of the practice often sets the tone for the management or operation function, or for retirement from active practice.

PRACTICE ADMINISTRATION

The second stage of the business cycle — the active management of the business — is as important in the practice of veterinary medicine as it is in a retail or manufacturing enterprise. It is in this cycle that the success or failure of the practice is determined.

Like law and medicine, veterinary medicine is a self-governing profession. Provincial regulatory bodies made up, for the most part, of other veterinarians, have the authority to license, discipline, and otherwise govern the profession. Provincial legislation regulates the operation of the practice according to uniform standards by establishing an objective standard to which a practitioner must adhere. In this manner the public is protected from unskilled and unethical practitioners. The rules that govern the veterinary profession vary somewhat from province to province. A list of the provincial statutes is set out in appendix D. In addition to the statutes themselves, veterinary practice is governed by regulations or bylaws passed pursuant to the legislation, which contain detailed rules covering the operation of a practice.

Failure to abide by the provisions of the legislation can result in disciplinary action by the provincial governing body. A list of the governing bodies is set out in appendix E. The governing bodies regulate the veterinary profession with the protection of the public in mind; in addition, most act as advocacy groups for the profession. The practitioner should be familiar with the provincial legislation, and should manage his or her practice with a view to maintaining compliance with all legal rules and regulations.

In Manitoba, the regulation of the veterinary profession is set out in the Veterinary Medical Act and the bylaws of the Manitoba Veterinary Medical Association. Among other things, the association has the power to prescribe requirements for membership, standards of practice, and codes of ethics. The association's powers extend to the setting of standards for employment of veterinary technicians. The Council of Management is made up of the immediate past president of the association and at least six other members.

PRACTICE POINT

The mandate of the provincial associations is primarily to promote the profession and protect the public interest. The veterinarian member of a provincial body must be aware of the public interest component of the regulatory body and recognize the perspective that it necessarily has in ensuring that adequate practice standards are met for the purpose of public protection.

In Nova Scotia, veterinarians are governed by the Veterinary Medical Act. The provincial regulatory body is the Nova Scotia Veterinary Medical Association, which delegates much of its administrative and disciplinary matters to the council of the association. The council is made up of the four officers of the association (president, vice-president, past president, and secretary-registrar), three executive members elected by the general membership, and one person appointed by the Canadian Veterinary Medical Association. Much of the detailed information required by the practitioner in Nova Scotia is contained in the association's bylaws.

In New Brunswick, the profession is regulated by a council of the New Brunswick Veterinary Medical Association. Section 4 of the New Brunswick Veterinarians Act provides that the council is to be made up of no fewer than six councillors, who shall "control, govern and manage, or supervise the control, government and management of the business and affairs of the Association and all aspects of the practice of veterinary medicine."

In Quebec, the law that governs the profession is different in form from that of the common law provinces. Nonetheless, the substance of the legislation is similar to the other provincial laws. The Quebec Professional Code covers most of the professions in the province: lawyers, doctors, dentists, architects, engineers, and, veterinarians. Schedule I of the Code includes the Corporation professionelle des médecins vétérinaires du Québec, the provincial regulatory body. According to section 2 of the

Code, the laws set out therein apply to all professional corporations; thus, one finds general rules for regulating the professions, which are supplemented by regulations under the Professional Code. The Office des professions du Québec has a duty to ensure that each professional organization adopts a code of ethics. Any regulations adopted by the office must be submitted to the Legislative Assembly of Quebec for approval prior to their adoption. The veterinarian in Quebec is also governed by an Interprofessional Council consisting of a member of each of the professional corporations listed in the Code. The Interprofessional Council may study and seek solutions to problems of a general nature encountered by the various professions. By section 23 of the Professional Code, the principal function of the veterinary organization is to ensure the protection of the public. To this end, the body is charged with supervising the practice of the profession by its members. Instead of a council, veterinarians are governed by a Bureau consisting of varying numbers of directors, depending on the number of members in the profession. By section 86 of the Code, the Bureau must, by resolution, keep an up-to-date roll of members. In addition, the Bureau must organize refresher courses and fix amounts of annual dues and levies.

In the discussions that follow, the Ontario statute will be used as the model; the general principles of the statute are similar to those of the other provinces. The full texts of the Ontario statute and regulations are set out in appendixes F and G.

LICENSING

Every student of veterinary medicine must become qualified in order to practice. Section 3(1) of the Ontario Veterinarians Act (VA) dictates that the College of Veterinarians of Ontario (CVO) is obligated to regulate the practice of veterinary medicine in Ontario and to govern its members in accordance with the VA. Further, the CVO is empowered to "establish, maintain and develop standards of qualification and standards of practice for the practice of veterinary medicine." The governing body of the CVO is the council of the college, which, by section 4 of the VA, is also the board of directors. The council is mandated to manage and administer the affairs of the college. By section 7 of the VA, the council has, subject to the approval of the Ontario cabinet, the power to make regulations relating to a number of matters, including the qualifications and requirements for the issuance of licences. Similar provisions are found in the Alberta legislation in section 13, which gives the council in that province the power to regulate all aspects of the profession. The legislation of most provinces creates a mandated council to govern the affairs of the provincial veterinary association.

A number of different types of licences are available to the veterinarian in Ontario. In general, every veterinarian with any form of licence must be a Canadian citizen or permanent resident, and must have completed to the satisfaction of the CVO tests indicating a proficiency in English-language skills (unless the applicant's primary and secondary school education or undergraduate veterinary training was conducted in English or French). The applicant must also complete a form of application and submit it to the registrar of the CVO. In addition, all licences are issued subject to the applicant's providing evidence that he or she has not been found guilty of professional misconduct, gross neglect, or impairment (discussed in chapter 11), and paying the prescribed fee to the CVO. In addition to these general rules, the applicant must also meet the requirements for the type of licence applied for.

The licensing of practitioners in Newfoundland and Labrador is delegated to the Newfoundland and Labrador Veterinary Licensing Board, which has the authority to examine all degrees, diplomas, and licences of any proposed member and to conduct examinations to ascertain the qualifications of persons to be registered. The board may, with the approval of the minister of forestry and agriculture in Newfoundland, make regulations prescribing the qualifications for registration, providing examinations, and exempting persons from examination. In addition, the board is given the express authority to provide a "code of ethics for practitioners of veterinary science." The board in Newfoundland and Labrador fulfils the same function as the council in other provinces.

The governing body in Prince Edward Island is the Prince Edward Island Veterinary Medical Association. The association, in turn, delegates authority to govern to a council pursuant to section 3.1 of the bylaws of the association. Any person who wishes to practise veterinary medicine in the province must first obtain a licence from the licensing board, which is made up of the council members (four officers and three other members) and not more than two members of the general public appointed by the lieutenant-governor in council. Any examinations required by the licensing board are set out in the bylaws, which vary according to the type of licence requested.

The Professional Code of Quebec states that no one may claim to be a veterinary surgeon or use any title that may lead to the belief that he or she holds a "valid, appropriate permit and is entered on the roll of the corporation empowered to issue the permit."

A helpful provision for out-of-province veterinarians is contained in the Veterinary Medical Act of Manitoba, which provides that the legislation does not prohibit a lawfully qualified practitioner from outside Manitoba to meet with a Manitoba veterinarian for consultation purposes.

The types of licences granted by the CVO are determined by sections 5 through 9 of the regulations to the VA. Each type of licence has a number of requirements that must be met in addition to the general licensing rules set out above. It is important to remember that the licence to practise is a privilege granted to successful applicants; it permits them to practise in the veterinary profession only so long as the CVO is satisfied that the holder of the licence is competent and complies with the legislation and regulations.

In Ontario, five types of licences are available: general, academic, public service, short-term, and educational. Each of these types of licences may be issued by the CVO subject to restrictions determined by the CVO. The veterinarian's practice can be continued only in accordance with those restrictions and conditions.

PRACTICE POINT

As a matter of law a licence is mere permission to engage in a certain activity. In a veterinary context, the provincial government grants the right to issue a licence to the regulatory body, which in turn must ensure that the terms of the licence are adhered to. You should remember that the licence to practice is a privilege that may be revoked; it is not a right.

The most popular licence is a general licence to operate a private clinic, either as an owner or as an employee of a practice. The requirements of a general licence include the possession of a basic degree from a recognized veterinary school, the passing of a national board test as set out by the American Veterinary Association, and the successful completion of a local examination. In certain circumstances the holder of a veterinary degree from an unaccredited veterinary school may be issued a licence if he or she successfully completes a clinical proficiency exam set by the Canadian Veterinary Medical Association.

An academic licence is granted to those who hold a veterinary degree and a full-time teaching or research appointment of professional rank at the Ontario Veterinary College of the University of Guelph. The applicant must complete the local examination. The holder of an academic licence may practise veterinary medicine only in the department in which the professional appointment has been made. This type of licence terminates automatically when the academic appointment ends.

Veterinarians employed by the federal government who have earned their veterinary degree from a recognized institution may apply for and be granted a public service licence. Like the academic licence-holder, the holder of a public service licence is restricted to practice that is in the course of his or her employment. The licence terminates when the employment ends. A typical public service licence holder is a federal meat inspector.

Short-term licences are issued to applicants who hold a degree in veterinary medicine and provide a written undertaking from another member of the CVO who is willing to supervise the applicant and continue to be responsible for the applicant after the licensee leaves Ontario. In addition, the applicant must be appointed by the CVO or a recognized group of veterinarians, or have the consent of the CVO, to perform specific veterinary services solely for a short term and special purpose. The short-term licence terminates on the earliest of the day on which the appointment of consent terminates, the day the holder of the licence leaves Ontario, and thirty days after the licence is issued.

An educational licence may be issued to the holder of a veterinary degree who is enrolled in postgraduate study at the OVC. This type of licence permits the applicant to practise only as may be required by the program of study and only under the supervision of a general licence holder employed by the University of Guelph. The educational licensee may receive remuneration only in the form of a fixed fee or a stipend. The licence terminates when the holder ceases to be enrolled in the course of study.

In Prince Edward Island, a jurisdiction that also has a veterinary school, the Atlantic Veterinary College, six different types of licences can be granted: a general licence to carry on clinical veterinary medicine activities in the province; a limited licence to carry on a practice limited to one or more species; an academic licence to practise at the Atlantic Veterinary College; an educational licence permitting the holder to practise in connection with an appointment as an intern or resident of the Atlantic Veterinary College; a short-term licence issued for up to six months; and an interim licence for those who have applied for one of the other licences and are awaiting its issuance. This last licence is valid for the lesser of ninety days or the next time at which the licensing board meets.

FACILITIES

In addition to setting out the types of licences that may be held by a veterinarian, the council of the CVO has the power to deal with all matters relating to the issuance, renewal, suspension, and revocation of certificates of accreditation for the operation of various types of veterinary facilities. Once again, the regulations under the VA dictate the rules relating to the types of veterinary facilities in which a licence holder may practice his or her profession.

Generally, every applicant for an accredited facility must submit the proper application form to the registrar of the CVO and pay the requisite fee. In addition, each applicant must provide a written undertaking to the CVO to be responsible for the facility, and must be an owner or partner in the practice that is to be conducted from the facility. Each applicant must be a general licence-holder or the holder of a restricted licence that is consistent with the type of practice set out in the accreditation.

The Prince Edward Island legislation, and in particular the bylaws of the province's Veterinary Medical Association, sets out detailed standards for veterinary facilities in that province. Bylaw 19 specifies the minimum standards to be met. The premises must be of "good construction and permanent in nature" and "neat, clean and in good repair and the facility shall be adequately heated, lighted, ventilated and screened." Signs and letterhead must conform to the ethical standards of the association. The practitioner's library must include a current edition of the provincial legislation and bylaws and adequate reference materials. These minimum standards are supplemented by additional rules according to the type of facility; for instance, a basic hospital facility must be constructed of water-impervious materials and be well drained. Hospitalized animals must be seen at least twice daily by a professional staff member and be kept under regular observation by lay staff during the working day. In a small-animal practice, the facilities must have separate rooms for examination and treatment, surgery, and private hospitalization, and a waiting room. Motor vehicles used in the practice (primarily large-animal practices) must be clean and in good repair. Clean overalls must be available for each call outside a hospital, and footwear must be cleaned and disinfected in the facilities after each call.

The standards for veterinary facilities are laid out in the bylaws of the Nova Scotia Veterinary Medical Association. Under the heading "Hospital and Practice Standards," the bylaws provide for the accreditation of several different types of facilities, including a small-animal house call practice and an animal medical centre. The former is a practice conducted from any vehicle used in a practice for the purpose of visits to a client's residence to examine and treat companion animals; the latter is an animal hospital that provides full and complete consultation, clinical, and hospital services by a licensed staff of veterinary scientists who are fully accredited to perform scientific research and conduct advanced education programs. The Nova Scotia legislation, which has some of the most detailed provisions in Canada, sets out a number of practice standards relating to records, reception, and restroom facilities, examination facilities, pharmacies, and libraries. It is mandatory that a copy of the provincial act and bylaws be included in the library of an accredited facility. The equipment necessary to conduct radiology, major surgical procedures, and non-surgical or dentistry functions is listed in the bylaws. Overnight compartments must have proper bedding and a method of being securely locked. Exercise runs must be at least fifteen square feet and two and one-half feet wide, with solid partitions of at least four feet in height.

In New Brunswick, the bylaws of the New Brunswick Veterinary Medical Association appear to dictate minimum practice facility standards for companion animal practices.

Practitioners in British Columbia are well served by the bylaws of their provincial association, in that it publishes a form of practice inspection report in appendix B to the bylaws of the association. This comprehensive form sets out in checklist fashion the standards required for a veterinary facility, and can serve as a benchmark by which the practitioner can conduct his or her own inspection before a visit from an appointed inspector (which situation can arise from a client complaint).

The Veterinary Medical Board of Manitoba has the power to enter, during reasonable hours, any premises in which veterinary medicine is being practised to determine whether or not the standards are being maintained.

At present, twelve different classes of veterinary facilities are listed in section 11 of Ontario regulation 1093 and its amendments: companion animal hospital, companion animal office, companion animal mobile office, companion animal mobile, companion animal emergency clinic, companion animal spay-neuter clinic, food-producing animal hospital, food-producing animal mobile, equine clinic, equine mobile, poultry service, and equine emergency mobile. To more clearly differentiate among types of clinics, the term "companion animal" is deemed not to include horses.

In Alberta we find four broad categories of facilities in the general regulations to the Alberta Veterinary Profession Act: ambulatory, house call, or consultation; clinic; hospital; and emergency clinic.

Generally, in all classes of facilities the certificate of accreditation expires three or five years after issuance: the former date applies when a facility has undergone an inspection by the CVO and deficiencies have been noted, and the latter when no deficiencies have been noted after inspection. In certain circumstances the accreditation expires earlier if a stationary practice is relocated or if any of the general requirements for accreditation are not met.

CERTIFICATES

The accreditation of a facility is evidenced by the issuance of a certificate by the CVO. With the exception of the mobile classes of accreditation, the certificate must be conspicuously displayed in the facility.

The various classes of accreditation have been established to regulate the type of practice carried on in the premises. For example, a companion animal certificate restricts the practitioner to the treatment of companion animals, just as a food-producing certificate restricts him or her to the treatment of food-producing animals and horses. The treatment of horses can take place only in premises that have an equine or food-producing accreditation.

Other restrictions are placed on various types of companion animal facilities. The veterinary services provided in a companion animal office cannot include radiology, major surgery, overnight confinement, or hospitalization. A companion animal hospital accreditation includes but is not restricted to those services. A companion animal mobile accreditation is specifically limited to a number of catalogued treatments, including assessments, vaccinations, sedation, surgical repair of simple wounds, nail clipping, minor dental treatment, collection of semen, and artificial insemination.

Emergency clinics for companion animals must have a veterinarian on duty in the facility, and that veterinarian must be reasonably available for service every weekday from at least 7:00 p.m. to 9:00 a.m. the following day, every weekend from 7:00 p.m. Friday until 9:00 a.m. the following

Monday, and every statutory holiday from 7:00 p.m. on the day preceding the holiday to 9:00 a.m. the day after the holiday.

In Prince Edward Island, every licensed veterinarian is required to ensure twenty-four-hour emergency service within the limits of his or her particular licence. If emergency service is to be provided by a colleague licensee, written verification of such an affiliation may be requested by the licensing board of the province. Failure to comply with these provisions could result in suspension from practice.

A spay-neuter companion animal clinic is restricted to spay and neuter procedures, including pre-, intra-, and postoperative care.

RECORDS MANAGEMENT

It should not be surprising that there are exacting requirements for recordkeeping in any veterinary facility. Accurate documentation of presentation, diagnosis, and treatment notes is required by the profession and the public. The records for companion animals must contain some form of patient identification, species, age, and sex. In addition, the records must include the client's name, address, and telephone numbers. An emergency contact person, together with all other relevant communication data, must be set out in the event that the owner is likely to be absent from his or her residence while the animal is confined. The date of each visit, together with an accurate history of the animal's health, including vaccinations and weight, must be maintained. The particulars of assessment and any professional advice given to the client must also be noted. Any medical or surgical treatment must be recorded, including the name, strength, dose, and quantity of any drug dispensed. The fees charged for the services and the final assessment of the animal must also be recorded.

Similar requirements for recordkeeping apply to poultry and food-producing facilities.

The requirements for recordkeeping are similar in Quebec, and are set out in the regulations to the Quebec Professional Code and the Veterinary Surgeons Act.

All records must be legibly written or typewritten, kept in a systematic order (either alphabetically or chronologically) and, in Ontario, retained for at least five years after the date of the last entry in the record or for at least two years after the veterinarian ceases practice. Records may be maintained in any electronic medium, such as a computer disk, provided that the information can be printed promptly and that any changes in the recorded information are clearly indicated as changes.

Accurate records can mean the difference between success or failure in any disciplinary or liability proceeding; accordingly, the astute practitioner will treat records management meticulously.

PRACTICE POINT

Quite apart from the legal requirement to maintain accurate records, it is only good practice management to establish good recordkeeping habits. Should a legal difficulty arise in the future, the availability of documentary evidence is often essential to success. You should develop a set of standard forms of records to ensure that your recordkeeping habits permit you to document your practice activities easily, quickly, and without undue administrative burdens.

ADMINISTRATION OF DRUGS

Apart from the technical records required in practice, separate rules govern the recordkeeping relating to the use and dispensing of drugs in a practice. These records must be legible and may be recorded electronically.

Every veterinarian in Ontario who dispenses drugs must maintain a systematic method for filing the records required. Upon the acquisition of a supply of a drug, the veterinarian must immediately record the date of purchase, the name, strength, and quantity of the drug, the name and address of the supplier, the purchase price, and, in the case of a controlled drug or narcotic, the signature of the veterinarian who made the purchase. Similar requirements are found in British Columbia in the practice inspection form, schedule B to the bylaws of the British Columbia Veterinary Medical Association. Bylaw 21 of the New Brunswick Veterinary Medical Association governs the documentation relating to the dispensing of drugs. If drug treatment is required but the veterinarian does not have a dispensary, a written prescription must be provided to the client or an oral prescription to the pharmacist of the client's choice.

Additional rules govern the operation of a drug dispensary. These records must include the name and address of the owner of the animal for which the drug was dispensed, the name, strength, and quantity of drug, the directions for use (if different from a manufacturer's label), the date of dispensing, and the price charged. These records must be maintained for at least five years or until the veterinarian ceases practice. Similar requirements are set out for the labelling of containers in which drugs are held and given to the client, subject to certain exceptions.

The dispensing of controlled drugs and narcotics must also be recorded. In addition, these types of drugs must be protected against loss or theft. In the event of a loss or theft, the veterinarian has a statutory obligation to report the occurrence to the police immediately and within ten days to the federal minister of health and welfare. Lay staff are prohibited from dealing with controlled or narcotic drugs; only a licensed veterinarian may deal with them. The drugs must be stored in a locked cabinet.

Similar rules for poisons are set out, including a requirement that the container be marked legibly and conspicuously with the word "POISON."

Finally, other rules govern the labelling of containers for certain drugs listed in the regulations, and the dispensing of those drugs in child-resistant packages in ordinary circumstances.

A veterinarian may not administer, dispense, or prescribe a drug unless he or she has assumed responsibility for making medical judgments relating to the animal, has a sufficient knowledge of the health history of the animal, and has conducted either a physical examination or another medically appropriate investigation so as to reach a general diagnosis. The veterinarian must believe that the drug is prophylactically or therapeutically necessary for the animal, and must be available in the event that contraindications appear.

No veterinarian can sign a blank prescription form or dispense a drug for resale except to another veterinarian or to a pharmacist. No drug can be dispensed from any facility other than the facility in which the veterinarian regularly practises.

Bylaw 21 of the New Brunswick Veterinary Medical Association sets out similar rules relating to the handling and dispensing of drugs. The demands for recordkeeping are detailed in bylaw 21.03, and include the name and address of the owner, the name, strength, and quantity of the drug dispensed, the directions for use, the date, the price, and the withholding times used in food-producing animals. Those records must be maintained for at least two years. Requirements for the dispensing of drugs in child-resistant containers are set out in the New Brunswick legislation.

The general rules for prescribing drugs in Quebec is set out in the regulations under the Professional Code and the Veterinary Surgeons Act of that province. Every prescription must be in writing, except in the case of an emergency. In the event that an oral prescription is given to anyone other than a pharmacist, a written prescription must be completed within forty-eight hours.

ADVERTISING

In today's economic climate, it is necessary to introduce effective marketing concepts in order to ensure the success of any commercial enterprise. However, like other professionals, veterinarians are restricted by law in the type and content of their advertising. These restrictions apply not only to · the professional practice of veterinary medicine, but also to ancillary services such as grooming and pet food sales.

PRACTICE POINT

Effective advertising is only one element of a marketing strategy. You should ensure that the content of any ad adheres strictly to the rules set out in the legislation; if in doubt, submit a proposed advertisement to your provincial association for their comments.

The regulations under the Ontario Veterinarians Act have recently been amended to permit advertising. There is a general prohibition on any form of advertising, announcement, or similar form of communication relating to professional or ancillary services except as specifically provided in the regulations themselves. The rules specify the type and content of permitted advertising. In Nova Scotia, detailed advertising rules are set out in a part of the legislation relating to ethical conduct; many provinces deal with advertising issues in this manner. Advertising is discussed in more detail in chapter 13.

Any veterinarian in Ontario may advertise, provided that the content of the ad is "factual, accurate and verifiable information that a reasonable person would consider relevant in the choice of a veterinarian." That information cannot be false, misleading or deceptive, must be readily comprehensible, and must contain no testimonial or comparative statements. The most difficult aspect of the rules is that the ad must be "dignified and in good taste." (No objective test for dignity and good taste is set out.) The ad cannot contain any information about fees or any reference to a specific drug or other therapeutic treatment.

Advertising of fees is limited to that which is displayed inside the veterinary facility. The display must be of a size and in a location such that it cannot be read from outside the facility.

Many new clients are referred to a practice by another happy client. Section 38 of the Ontario regulations specifically prohibits any member from directly or indirectly participating in a system whereby clients are steered or recommended to the practitioner by another practitioner. The obvious exception to this rule is that which permits a practitioner to refer a client to a veterinary specialist.

Veterinarians often participate in other associated businesses such as the development of pet foods and supplies. These types of activities are addressed in the legislation. Veterinarians are prohibited from causing or permitting their names to appear in any advertising offering to the public any product or service other than his or her professional services. Presumably, product endorsements fall within this prohibition. Veterinarians may be associated with the advertising of services or products in any publication that is intended to be read principally by veterinarians. In addition, a scholarly article on the relative merits of a particular product or service would be permitted.

PRACTICE POINT

The best and most effective form of advertising and promotion is the recommendation of a happy client. You should always strive to provide the best service to every client; however, from time to time, notwithstanding your best efforts a client is not happy and launches a campaign to discredit you. In a legal sense, you are entitled to take active steps against any attempt to defame you, pursuant to the laws of libel and slander; however, you should be aware that there are very strict time limits within which you must act in order to preserve your legal rights.

Promotional advertising is restricted by a general prohibition on the veterinarian's ability to communicate with or attempt to communicate with any person in order to solicit patronage for a clinic or any ancillary services. This would suggest that any indiscriminate distribution of a brochure or pamphlet is not permissible. However, such communications — provided that they fall within the general guidelines respecting "good taste" — may be sent to those members of the public who would find the availability of such services useful. Any such communication must be clearly marked "advertisement" on each page. In addition, the practitioner may distribute to regular clients general information about animal health, preventive medicine, or recent developments in veterinary science. A form of tickler system may be instituted in the practice to contact regular clients when health maintenance procedures are due to be carried out. In these cases a "regular client" is any person who uses the professional services of the practice regularly and with reasonable frequency, and who has not requested a transfer of records to another veterinary clinic. A client who engages the services of an employee veterinarian is deemed to be a client of the owner.

Particularly if you are buying a practice as a going concern, the name of the practice and its associated goodwill can be an important element in marketing and advertising. In addition to the general rules relating to names of accredited facilities discussed above, further rules are set out in the regulations. In Ontario, the practice name must be registered with the cvo. The registered name is the only one under which a veterinarian can practise. The name of the facility may be chosen by the professional, subject to the approval of the Accreditation Committee of the cvo. The name must contain a geographical reference appropriate to the location of the facility, or the surname of a member who is or was associated with the practice. In addition, the name must contain the word "animal," "pet," or "veterinary," unless the practice is restricted to a single species, in which case the name of that species, one of the key words, or both must appear. If the practice is restricted to poultry, the word "poultry," with or without the word "veterinary," must appear. A name will not be approved by the Accreditation Committee if these rules are not satisfied, if the name is, in their opinion, unfitting or improper, or if the name is likely to be confused with the name of another facility. Any name that was in use before November 16, 1985 and conforms to the other rules need not be referred to the committee for approval prior to continuing its use. This is an important consideration if you are thinking of purchasing an existing practice.

Similarly, the New Brunswick Veterinarians Act provides that the name of the practice may contain a geographic reference appropriate to the location of the facility, and the word "animal," "pet," or "veterinary," unless the practice is restricted to a particular species, in which case the name of the species and one of the foregoing words can be used. The bylaws of the New Brunswick Veterinary Medical Association provide that the name of a practice cannot conflict or be confused with the designation of any other veterinary facility.

The proper use of the words permitted in a facility name was at issue in 1985 in Ontario when the Ontario Veterinary Association (now the CVO) found one of its members guilty of professional misconduct when the name "Animal Hospital of Oakville" was used by the veterinarian. In *Cormack v. Ontario Veterinary Association* (7 OAC 159) the veterinarian sought a judicial review of the finding of professional misconduct. The Ontario Divisional Court held that while the legislation in Ontario dictated the words that could be used in the name of a practice, the rules did not state any particular order of the words. The court found that there was no need for the three elements to appear in a specific order. The veterinarian's suspension was reversed.

PERSONNEL PLANNING

One of the fastest-growing areas of commercial litigation in Canada is employment law. Like other professionals, the veterinary practitioner requires some knowledge of the rights of the employer and the employee so as to avoid lengthy and expensive lawsuits. Often, conflicts can be avoided through the use of properly drafted employment contracts for associate veterinarians, locums, or lay staff, which clearly set out the terms of employment. In this part of the chapter we will look at the provincial employment standards acts and the doctrine of wrongful dismissal.

PRACTICE POINT

Your employees can be your most valuable asset or your greatest liability. As in any legal relationship, the employer should seek to achieve certainty in the work environment.

THE EMPLOYMENT RELATIONSHIP

The English common law of "master and servant" forms the basis for modern employment law. At common law, judges determined that a "contract of service" was essential to the employment relationship. Thus, an employee is defined as a person who provides service to an employer and is under the direct control of the employer. An employee is not an independent contractor. That latter designation refers to a person who enters into a contractual relationship with another to complete a specific task, usually within a specific time and for an agreed-upon price. No continuing relationship exists after the task is completed. The distinction can be crucial. Only an employee can initiate a wrongful dismissal action, for example, and an independent contractor is normally entitled to certain business tax deductions not available to an employee. Remember that professionals as well as lay staff can be either employees or independent contractors.

PRACTICE POINT

Sometimes you may prefer to engage an independent contractor rather than an employee — for example, to assist with a particular patient or to relieve a particularly heavy workload in your practice. For management purposes you must know which relationship exists between you and your personnel.

Over the years the courts have established a number of tests to determine whether an individual is an employee or an independent contractor:

1. **Degree of control:** to the extent that the principal exercises a high degree of control over the day-to-day actions of another veterinarian, it is likely that the veterinarian is an employee.

2. **Ownership of tools and equipment:** generally speaking, independent contractors own their own tools and veterinary aids.

3. **Risk of profit and loss:** employees generally do not share in the profits and losses of the practice.

4. **Manner and consistency of payment:** regular payments, subject to statutory deductions and withholding tax, are indicative of employment rather than independent engagement.

Notwithstanding any written contract that the parties have entered into that refers to one party as an "employee" or an "independent contractor," the courts will employ the tests set out above and come to their own determination of the true nature of the relationship.

The employer-employee relationship may be created either orally or in writing by the formation of a contract. As well, the relationship may be implied from the behaviour and conduct of the parties.

THE EMPLOYMENT CONTRACT

To provide the greatest amount of certainty for the employer and the employee, it is recommended that a properly drafted employment contract be entered into by the parties. A contract permits the veterinarian employer the opportunity to change the common law relationship that would otherwise exist so that it reflects the actual expectations of the parties.

PRACTICE POINT

Given the plethora of employment law issues, it is strongly recommended that a formal written employment contract or letter of agreement be made a part of your practice management. Certainty in the relationship will promote greater trust and loyalty between the veterinarian and his or her staff.

The employment contract can be as comprehensive as the parties desire. A typical contract will deal with the following issues:

1. **The length of the relationship:** It is usually a good idea to provide that the relationship will be for a specified period of time, which may be renewed.

2. **Compensation and bonuses:** This section of the contract establishes the amount of payment for services rendered. For tax purposes, you should ensure that all necessary statutory deductions and withholdings are made. Incentives may be provided to employees through a bonus program based on new clients introduced to the hospital or other revenue-generating or cost-saving practices.

3. **Method of remuneration:** Specify whether cheques are to be issued weekly, biweekly, or monthly.

4. **Job descriptions and responsibilities:** A carefully thought out description of the employee's duties will prove helpful in the event that the employee is found to have breached the employment contract.

5. **Holidays and excused absences:** The efficiency of office administration is improved if each employee knows the conditions of holidays, vacations, and sick leave.

6. **Workplace rules and safety:** The manner in which you wish to see your clinic operate and policies for occupational safety can be set out. Breach of these rules may be sufficient cause for termination.

7. **Confidentiality:** The veterinary code of ethics in each province dictates the need for confidentiality and privacy for your clients. A breach of confidence not only compromises your professional services but is also likely to result in detrimental public relations for your hospital.

8. **Terminations:** This provision should specify what constitutes a termination of the relationship and any notice provisions. Provision for the return of records and equipment to the hospital should also be dealt with.

9. **Non-competition covenants:** A valued associate will quickly start to attract regular clients. Upon termination of the employment relationship, the prudent owner will rely on a form of non-competition agreement to protect his or her market territory. Such an agreement, to be lawfully enforceable, must be reasonably restricted in duration and territory.

10. **Hours of work:** For some employees, particularly part-time employees, it is important to specify the hours that they are expected to be on duty.

Through an employment contract, the parties can specify the terms of the relationship at a time when no disputes exist between them and consensus can be reached. If no contract is signed, the parties will be left to the common law and the court system. Like many other commercial agreements, the employment contract can be an effective policing tool to avoid potential problems.

In a veterinary context, the enforceability of a non-competition covenant was the issue presented to the Manitoba Court of Appeal in 1992 in *Friesen and Hamilton v. McKague* ([1993] 1 WWR 627). The court reviewed the terms of an agreement which contained a provision that, upon termination of the agreement for any reason, the former employee could not practise veterinary medicine in any manner for three years within twenty-five miles of the clinic. The contract was to continue until June 30, 1991. On June 3, 1991, the practitioner left his employment and leased space to open his own practice within the restricted area. The Court of Appeal reviewed the lower court's decision, and cited the case law to the effect that such covenants are generally unenforceable; however, if the employer shows that it had a legitimate business interest to protect and that the restraint was reasonable, both as between the parties and in the public interest, then it may be enforced. Restrictive clauses that contain "blanket" restrictions are generally not enforceable; in this case, however, all parties had received legal advice before they entered into the agreement, and the employer showed that it had a legitimate business interest to protect. The court found that the restriction was reasonable.

COMMON LAW DUTIES OF THE PARTIES

As previously mentioned, the employer and employee are each subject to the duties set out in the case law. Among other things, the employee must obey lawful orders, exercise care and skill, exercise good faith, account to the employer in financial matters, and not divulge confidential information. Similarly, employers must provide a safe workplace, supply the equipment necessary to perform the job, and reimburse the employee for expenses properly incurred for the benefit of the employer. Many common law duties have been enshrined in legislation, particularly those duties relating to health and safety in the workplace.

WRONGFUL DISMISSAL

Each year many suits alleging wrongful dismissal are filed in Canada. These actions are commenced by terminated employees who feel that they have been dismissed from their employment without adequate reason, adequate notice, or a payment of money in lieu of notice. In effect, the action is founded in breach of contract — that is, breach by the employer of the employment contract.

An employer is not liable for damages to an employee if the employee was terminated for just cause; in other words, the employer must have a legally recognized reason for terminating the contract. If just cause exists, then the employer may effect an immediate termination without notice or payment.

In Quebec, a similar form of wrongful dismissal doctrine exists. The Civil Code specifies relatively short notice periods for "domestic servants, journeymen and labourers" in article 1668; article 1027 appears to adopt principles of notice relating to usual and customary practices. It appears that employees with some management responsibility do not fall within the ambit of article 1668, and will therefore be entitled to reasonable notice determined in accordance with the length of their employment and the scope of their duties.

The onus is upon the employer to show that just cause for dismissal actually exists in a form that is recognized by the law. Just cause may be proved for any of the following reasons:

1. **Dishonesty:** An employee who lies about a client-related matter or steals goods or money from the practice can be dismissed without notice.

2. **Incompetence:** The determination of what conduct is "incompetent" is an important aspect of termination for this cause. An employee's incompetence should be documented in detail, together with written warnings issued before dismissal.

3. **Physical abuse:** Any assault by the employee on the employer, other employees, or clients will, in most cases, be grounds for dismissal. In a veterinary context the abuse of an animal by an employee would be so fundamentally at odds with the nature of the business as to constitute just cause for termination.

4. **Drunkenness:** Repeated intoxication while on the job is grounds for termination. Once again, written warnings should be issued.

5. **Conflict of interest:** Most employees will work only for one clinic at a time. In those cases, conflicts of interest should not arise. Professional staff are also governed by the provincial codes of ethics, which generally prohibit any form of conflict of interest.

6. **Insolence:** Disrespect to the employer or supervisors is not to be tolerated; a written warning should be issued before termination.

PRACTICE POINT

The prudent employer will conduct periodic reviews of employees' performance, and, in writing, point out weaknesses in performance that may eventually result in having just cause for dismissal. Without such written evidence, your ability to summarily dismiss an employee is prejudiced.

If no just cause exists for termination, the employer is bound to give adequate notice of termination or a payment in lieu of notice. In determining what is adequate notice, one must consider a number of factors: the age of the employee, the character of the job, the length of the employee's service, and the availability of alternative employment. As one would expect, as an employee grows older or serves for a longer period of time and gains more responsibility the required period of notice increases.

Do not fall into the trap of believing that the notice requirements set out in the provincial employment standards acts are necessarily adequate. Those provisions are generally minimum standards only, below which an employer cannot fall. At present, the Ontario rules require an employer to give one week's notice or payment in lieu of notice for each year of service, up to a maximum of eight weeks. In Manitoba, the Employment Standards Act provides that termination cannot be undertaken without notice, and states that the period between the date on which notice is given and the date of termination cannot be shorter than the period in respect of one regular instalment of wages or salary for the worker. In the event that the pay period is less frequent than monthly, the statute says only that "reasonable notice" must be given.

Unlawful termination may also occur in situations where the employer changes the nature of the job so dramatically that the employee may elect to treat the change as constructive dismissal, or the equivalent of firing. Demotions, reduction in salary, changes in benefits, or misconduct by the employer are all potential examples of constructive dismissal.

PROCEDURE FOR TERMINATION

The objective of the prudent employer is to avoid the wrongful dismissal action. Termination without just cause should be carried out in a termination interview, and the employee should be given a written letter of termination outlining reasonable proposals for payments in lieu of notice, and assistance in finding alternative employment through the engagement of employment counsellors and retraining services. A form of termination letter is set out in appendix H.

One of the best ways to avoid the problem of dismissal is through a properly drafted employment agreement (similar to those reproduced in appendixes I and J), which binds the parties to a specific plan in the event of termination of the employment relationship.

The employer is also required to provide the terminated employee with a separation certificate, which will enable the employee to claim unemployment insurance benefits.

PROVINCIAL EMPLOYMENT STANDARDS

The Ontario Employment Standards Act, the Manitoba Employment Standards Act, the Alberta Employment Standards Code, and the Labour Standards Codes of the Northwest Territories and Nova Scotia all establish certain minimum standards governing conditions of employment.

In Ontario, regulation 285(3) to the Employment Standards Act specifically excludes qualified veterinary practitioners from the employment standards relating to hours of work, minimum wages, overtime pay, statutory holidays, and paid vacation. Presumably, the rationale for this exclusion is that the nature of a professional calling necessitates the keeping of long and irregular hours. The material that follows relates primarily to the lay staff of a veterinary clinic, not to professional staff.

HOLIDAYS

In Ontario, an employer is obliged to grant every employee two weeks' vacation with pay upon the completion of each twelve months of employment. The amount of vacation pay must not be less than an amount equal to 4 percent of the employee's wages in the twelve months of employment for which the vacation is granted. The vacation period can be in one two-week block, or two one-week blocks; however, it must be taken not later than ten months after the end of the twelve- month period for which it was given. In Alberta, an employee with at least five years' service is entitled to at least three weeks' vacation. The rate of vacation pay also increases for longer term employees to 6 percent of the employees' wages in that province.

HOURS OF WORK

Except in some unusual circumstances, an employee in Ontario must not work more than eight hours per day and forty-eight hours per week. The Manitoba act dictates that the "standard hours" of work are forty in a week and eight in a day.

OVERTIME PAY

Except in some unusual circumstances, an Ontario employee who works more than forty-four hours in any week is to be paid, for each hour worked in excess of forty-four, overtime pay at an amount not less than one and one-half times the regular rate of pay. Identical provisions are contained in the Alberta and Nova Scotia acts.

PAY EQUITY

Section 32 of the Ontario Employment Standards Act states that no employer shall differentiate between male and female employees by paying a female at a rate of pay less than the rate paid to a male (or vice versa) for substantially the same kind of work performed in the same practice where the work requires substantially the same skill, effort, and responsibility. However, an employer can differentiate between male and female employees on the basis of seniority, merit, or a system that measures earnings by quantity or quality of production. Similarly, the Nova Scotia Labour Standards Code says that an employer cannot pay a female employee at a rate less than that paid to a male employee for substantially the same work. An employer may establish that a factor or factors other than gender justifies a different rate of wages, and in those circumstances will not breach the act. The onus is on the employer to establish the justifying factors.

MATERNITY LEAVE

An employer is prohibited from terminating an employee who is entitled in law to a leave of absence for maternity. However, the employer may require that the leave be taken at such time as the duties of her position cannot reasonably be performed by her, or the performance of her work is materially affected by the pregnancy. An employee who is pregnant and has been employed for at least thirteen weeks prior to the estimated date of delivery is entitled to a leave of absence of at least seventeen weeks. In Ontario, the employee is required to give at least two weeks' notice of the date upon which she intends to commence her leave of absence; in Manitoba four weeks' notice is required. A returning employee must be reinstated to her position by the employer or be provided with alternative work of a comparable type at not less than the wage earned at the time of her leave and without loss of seniority. In the Northwest Territories, the employee must provide four weeks' notice of maternity leave and, if requested, must provide the employer with a medical certificate confirming the pregnancy. The employee is then entitled to a leave of not more than twenty weeks, commencing any time during the period of eleven weeks prior to the expected delivery date. The Labour Standards Act permits the employee to request an extension of the leave without pay to a maximum of six weeks if the actual date of delivery is later than the anticipated date.

SUPERVISION OF STAFF

In some cases, the level of supervision of some staff members is referred to in legislation. In fact, some provinces establish special categories of membership in the professional veterinary association for such lay employees as veterinary technicians.

Specific employment rules are set out in the New Brunswick Veterinarians Act relating to the employment of "animal health auxiliaries." Bylaw 19 defines such an employee as one who holds a certificate or diploma from a school approved by the council of the New Brunswick Veterinary Medical Association; has met the educational requirements set out in the rules; has paid all required fees; and has his or her name entered on the register maintained by the provincial registrar. Auxiliaries are permitted to perform under the "direction and supervision" of a practising veterinarian those tasks and duties for which they have been trained and have been approved by the provincial council.

In Prince Edward Island, veterinary technicians may be subject to the Veterinary Profession Act through the ability of the Prince Edward Island Veterinary Medical Association to establish an ancillary body of technicians who, under the direction of a licensed practitioner, perform certain technical procedures. The council of the association is permitted to establish standards of training and qualifications for technicians and lay assistants. In addition, special rules are set out for "preceptors," who are licensed veterinarians who train undergraduate students in veterinary medicine. A student who has completed all but his or her final year of undergraduate study at an approved veterinary school and who is enrolled in the final year thereof may enter into the employment of a preceptor and perform veterinary services at or under the direction of the preceptor for a period not exceeding six months. That period of cooperative education may be extended with the approval of council. During the period of such employment, the preceptor is permitted to charge and collect fees for the services performed by the student.

The Nova Scotia Veterinary Medical Act contains provisions similar to those of Prince Edward Island relating to employment of students by a preceptor.

Section 24 of the bylaws of the Nova Scotia Veterinary Medical Association state that the veterinarian has an obligation to be physically present when supervising his or her assistants, and must attend on house or farm calls with the assistant. No assistant is permitted to make a diagnosis or determine a treatment.

In British Columbia, some of the activities of employees are dealt with in the bylaws of the British Columbia Veterinary Medical Association. While supervision in activities is assumed, the level of supervision for some activities is set out in the bylaws. For instance, radiographic procedures, collection of specimens, and administration of medications (except narcotics, vaccines, or controlled drugs) can be completed with indirect supervision. Direct supervision is required for monitoring anaesthetized patients, administering vaccines, cleaning and preparing surgical sites, and performing dental procedures other than dental surgery. Direct personal supervision is required if the employee is to induce and maintain anaesthesia, suture skin, or administer narcotics or controlled drugs.

In 1989, the Manitoba Court of Queen's Bench dealt with one aspect of the supervision of employees and delegation of work to them. In *Robelesky v. Veterinary Medical Board (Manitoba)* (60 Man. R. (2d) 15), a client brought a small dog to a clinic to have it immunized against rabies. A registered animal health technician employed at the clinic was on duty. The defendant veterinarian was not present, but had left a pre-signed blank certificate certifying that he had immunized the dog against rabies. The technician, while permitted to administer the vaccine pursuant to the by-laws of the Veterinary Medical Act of Manitoba, could not render any diagnoses. On appeal from a conviction of professional misconduct, the court confirmed the finding of the trial court. The court reasoned that good veterinary practice required a diagnosis of the health of a small animal prior to vaccination, which was wholly within the responsibility of the veterinarian and could not be delegated to an employee. The court found that by pre-signing the certificate to be used for any animal that might be brought to the clinic, the veterinarian was in breach of the rules of professional conduct.

This case serves as a good example of the damaging results that can flow from becoming too comfortable with good and talented employees in practice. In certain cases the veterinarian *must* be present to adequately supervise some procedures and perform others. Presumably, this case would be similarly determined in Quebec. Under that jurisdiction's Code of Ethics the practitioner must not give a diagnosis before personally inquiring about the living conditions of the animal and examining it.

PROFESSIONAL RELATIONS

Many veterinarians either practise in partnership or share an office with others. The reasons for doing so are varied: to enable the fostering of a specialty, to share the workload and financial burden of the practice, or merely to have someone to act as a sounding board for cases or issues about which one is unsure. The legal mechanisms for doing so are varied as well. Many people believe that the relationship between professionals is always that of a partnership; however, depending on how the relationship is established and maintained, it could be an ill-defined association, a co-tenancy, or a joint venture. You should know with certainty what kind of relationship you have with your colleagues. The legal consequences arising out of the relationship can easily lead to the success or failure of the practice.

PARTNERSHIP LAW

As discussed in chapter 1, when two or more persons, whether individuals or corporations, carry on business together with a view to profit, their relationship is called a partnership. The law recognizes two types of partnerships: the general partnership and the limited partnership. This discussion will focus on the more common general partnerships.

LIABILITY

In a general partnership the liability of each partner for the debts and other obligations of the partnership is unlimited; that is, each partner is responsible for the whole of the practice's liabilities. Unlike a corporation, a partnership is not a separate legal entity; therefore, the law governing the relationship of third parties — that is, patients and their owners - holds that each partner is the agent of the partnership and of the other partners when acting in the normal course of partnership business. In other words, the actions of one partner bind the other partners.

In keeping with the agency principles set out above, each partner is liable with the other partners to the full extent of their personal assets for all debts and obligations of the practice while engaged as a partner.

PRACTICE POINT

Given the litigious nature of our society, the prudent veterinarian will undertake appropriate judgment-proofing techniques before commencing practice in partnership so as to protect his or her personal assets from liabilities incurred by the partnership. For example, the practitioner could transfer his or her residence to a spouse as an effective way to insulate that significant asset. The use of a holding corporation which owns the assets of the practice is another good way to avoid problems.

Each partner's liability extends not only to contractual obligations, such as the lease of the professional premises, but to liability for negligence in the performance of duties.

FORMATION OF A PARTNERSHIP

For a partnership to exist, two or more individuals must carry on a business as defined under the legislation, with a view to profit. It could be suggested that, by law, you are mandated to pursue proper management techniques so as to ensure profit.

The existence of a partnership is defined by reference to the intention of the parties as disclosed by a written agreement or by the conduct of the parties. In each case, the courts will be looking for evidence that the definition of a partnership has been met. Without one of the three elements, no partnership exists.

> **PRACTICE POINT**
>
> To lend certainty to the relationship between colleagues and avoid any adverse business, liability, or tax consequences, the prudent veterinarian will arrange for a written partnership agreement to be prepared and signed. Recent court decisions have held that a written form of agreement is good evidence of the existence of the business relationship.

The complexity and the potential monetary value of your practice dictates that an informal, ill-defined relationship with other professionals is not helpful in establishing a strong and continuing practice.

BUSINESS NAMES

In Ontario, in the event that you wish to practise under a name other than your own personal name, the provisions of the Business Names Act must be complied with. A registration with the Ministry of Consumer and Commercial Relations must be filed, setting out the name of the enterprise, the names and addresses of the parties, and the signatures of the parties. The name cannot be the same as or deceptively similar to any other business name. A registration is valid for five years and may be renewed. Failure to register could result in a quasi-criminal prosecution and in the inability to maintain a lawsuit in Ontario. The cost of registration is minimal.

> **PRACTICE POINT**
>
> Immediately attend to the filing of the appropriate business name registration so as to avoid potential penalties.

In addition, provincial codes of ethics, regulations, and bylaws may impose other limitations on the name under which the partnership may carry on business. The Nova Scotia statute states that only a surname or a geographic reference, together with the words "veterinary," veterinarians," "veterinarian," "animal," "pet," or the name of a species, and "clinic," "hospital," or "services," and "housecall" can make up the name of your practice. Because Nova Scotia permits professional incorporation, the appropriate corporate identifier is also authorized — for example, "Ltd." or "Inc.".

TAXATION OF A PARTNERSHIP

In general, the income and losses of the business carried on in partnership are determined at the partnership level. Expenses, capital cost allowance, and other costs are deducted from the revenues of the partnership to determine whether the practice has a net income or a net loss. That income or loss is divided among the partners in proportion to their partnership interests, included in the calculation of net income and losses from other sources, and taxed at the individual partner's usual marginal rate.

PARTNER RELATIONS

The relationship between partners is the subject of provincial legislation known as the Partnerships Act in Ontario and in Manitoba. In the absence of a partnership agreement, the government will impute a set of rules to govern the relationship. For example, the Ontario legislation provides that the acts of any one partner bind all the other partners, and that all property brought into the partnership must be held and applied by the partners exclusively for the purposes of the partnership. Further, the statute sets out rules relating to partnership interests, and effectively states that all partners are entitled to share equally in the profits, take part in management, and resolve their differences by majority rule. Of particular significance is the fact that the partnership is dissolved on the death of a partner. In Alberta, similar provisions are contained in section 36 of the Partnership Act, which provides that the relationship is terminated on the death of a partner, subject to any agreement between the partners.

These rules are not usually acceptable to all partners in all situations, and they fail to deal with the unique aspects of a given practice. For example, you may not necessarily want all partners to have an equal ownership interest in the equipment necessary to carry on the practice.

PRACTICE POINT

Before determining whether you need a partnership agreement, famil-iarize yourself with the provisions of the Partnership Act in your province. In most instances, the legislated rules will not suit your rela-tionship; if this is the case, a written contract setting out the terms of the relationship between the partners should be prepared.

Because the legislative rules governing partner relations are likely to be inadequate for your practice, it is good business planning to draft your own partnership agreement. Such planning, undertaken at the outset of the relationship, will avoid the significant costs and delays associated with partnership disputes that must be resolved through the court system.

PARTNERSHIP AGREEMENTS

A sample partnership agreement is reproduced in appendix c. In those provinces where incorporation is permitted, a similar agreement may be entered into by the shareholders, which will contain virtually the same type of planning between co-owners of the practice. A typical agreement deals with the following matters, among others:

1. the distribution of partnership income between the partners and the quantum and regularity of such payments in terms of partnership draws against future profits;

2. contributions to capital equipment (initial contributions can be acknowledged and future requirements set out);

3. the name of the partnership and the ownership thereof (because the name can be of significant value on dissolution, it is important that the rights to and restrictions on the continued use of the name be clearly set out);

4. transfers of partnership interests, including transfers internally among existing partners and the ability of an existing partner to transfer an interest or a part thereof to an outsider;

5. admission and expulsion of partners (rules relating to the contributions, if any, of new partners who are elevated from associate status and the realignment of the partnership interests as a result of a new admission, as well as provision for future occurrences, such as the loss of one's licence to practise, which may be grounds for expulsion from the practice);

6. banking and financing arrangements, including the name of the bank and the names of those authorized to sign financial documents;

7. management responsibilities, such as the naming of a managing partner to look after the administrative and management functions of the practice;

8. disposition on the death of a partner and life insurance (you may wish to provide for policies of life insurance so that the remaining partners have the financial resources necessary to fund any potential purchase of the interest of a deceased partner from his or her estate);

9. retirement of a partner, including the age for retirement and the possible continuation in practice of the retiree as a consultant; and

10. dissolution and termination (the automatic or other termination of the partnership on the occurrence of a specific event).

The contents of a partnership agreement are limited only by the creativity and expertise of the parties involved and their professional advisers.

PRACTICE POINT

If you prepare a formal agreement for your professional partnership, each partner should seek independent legal and accounting advice concerning its contents and consequences. The success of your practice, now governed by a written contract, is threatened if any party to the agreement feels that he or she was not adequately represented or was unduly influenced in the preparation of the agreement.

Remember, to the extent that no other agreement exists, or is undeterminable owing to lack of evidence of conduct, the relationship between partners will be governed by legislation.

Finally, whether or not a formal partnership agreement exists, each partner is deemed to have a duty of trust to the other partners. This duty, known in law as a fiduciary duty, dictates that each partner must act in the best interests of the partnership and not in his or her own self-interest. To the extent that it can act as a policing tool for the honouring of this duty, the formal agreement plays an important role in practice management.

FINANCIAL PLANNING

Very often, the revenues generated by a new or expanded veterinary practice are not sufficient to meet the practice's cash-flow and debt-servicing needs, and it is necessary for the principals to acquire financing elsewhere, either privately or through an institutional lender. The growth and well-being of your practice depends on your relationship with your lender and your ability to obtain credit on reasonable terms. In this chapter we will discuss the various means of obtaining funds, and examine the purpose and nature of common security documents and negotiable instruments.

There are two main ways in which to obtain funds to expand your practice or consolidate other debts: equity financing and debt financing. Which method you choose will depend on the nature of your practice and your lender's requirements. Each method has its advantages and disadvantages.

EQUITY FINANCING

Equity financing gives the person or institution that lends the money the right to participate in the growth of the business. The regulations under most provincial veterinary legislation prohibit the equity participation in profits in a practice with anyone other than a partner who is also a veterinarian; therefore, it is unlikely that equity financing can be obtained other than from the personal resources of a partner. Through the sale of partnership units or shares in a corporation, funds are provided in exchange for the right to participate in the future growth and revenues of the practice. Partnership units can be transferred either publicly or privately; however, it is unlikely that there would be any public investment in a Canadian veterinary practice.

From the investor's point of view, the main advantage of equity financing is that he or she becomes one of the owners of the practice. From the borrower's point of view, this is often one of the main disadvantages, since it may result in loss of management control. However, equity ownership does not always require the repayment of funds on a regular basis to the investor, which can alleviate some cash-flow difficulties.

The most common type of equity financing involves the issuance of shares in a corporation. Most small businesses are incorporated as private corporations as defined in the provincial securities legislation, which imposes strict rules with respect to the issuing of securities. The Ontario Securities Act prohibits the issuing of a public invitation to purchase shares in a private corporation. Any transfers of shares to investors must be consented to by the directors of the corporation. In Ontario a prospectus must be issued, giving true and fair disclosure of all material facts relating to the investment if the corporation does not fall within the private company rules. (The public issue of shares in a corporation is an extremely expensive endeavour and not used, mainly for that reason, by small businesses.) The key question then becomes, who is "the public"? Provided that an invitation is not made to all persons, many cases have held that acquiring a third-party investor does not offend the Securities Act. As well, there are numerous exemptions from the prospectus requirement contained within the legislation. All of these rules have similar application for a partnership and the issuance of partnership units; it is unlikely that this type of financing would ever be sought for a veterinary practice.

DEBT FINANCING

The second and more common form of financing is debt financing. A practice may arrange a loan privately or through an institutional lender. Such loans have a fixed schedule of repayment of principal together with a fixed or variable rate of interest. The lender has no further immediate right to participate in the practice. Provided that the loaned funds are used for a proper business purpose, the interest component of any repayment is properly tax-deductible by the borrower. From the borrower's point of view, the obvious disadvantage of debt financing is that regular repayment is required and, if a variable interest rate is applicable, the maintenance cost of the loan can increase.

PRACTICE POINT

Develop a good relationship with your banker. Meet with him or her on a regular basis; explain the intricacies of veterinary practice so that he or she has a proper understanding of the nature of your practice. At law, your banker owes you a duty of trust and is obliged to provide you with sound advice. It is your responsibility to ensure that your banker has the knowledge necessary to render that advice.

Debt financing is the most common method of borrowing in veterinary practices; the remainder of this discussion will concentrate on the forms of debt instruments and the means by which the lender secures the debt.

DUTIES OF THE INSTITUTIONAL LENDER

FIDUCIARY DUTY

The courts have found that an institutional lender — whether a bank, an insurance company, a brokerage firm, or a trust company — and its employees act in a fiduciary capacity in relation to their customers. This means that the lender must act in utmost good faith. This position of trust becomes very important in terms of the advice and counselling provided by the lender's employees, who must be completely open and "up front" with respect to the form of loan arrangement, the costs thereof, and the circumstances that will bring the loan into default.

CONFIDENTIALITY

Courts have ruled that banks are bound by a strict code of confidentiality. This means that the lender cannot discuss your business affairs with any unauthorized party without your consent.

BUSINESS PLANS

A written business plan is very useful when you apply to an institutional lender for credit. More important, a formal plan, which is essentially a statement of projected profits and losses, provides you with benchmarks against which you can conduct your own analysis of how your clinic is performing. Projections and targets for fees billed, together with a realistic outline of the expenses to be incurred, is of fundamental importance to you and your lender in assessing your creditworthiness. Business plans are often prepared on a five-year basis, and should be reviewed at least annually and adjusted to fit changing circumstances. A sample business plan checklist is found in appendix K.

The credit manager who handles your account will be better disposed to assist you if he or she feels confident that you know about the financial status of your practice, and where it stands in the community vis-à-vis your competitors. The presentation of a business plan is a reasonable requirement of the banks and other financial institutions to assist them in providing terms of credit while helping you to manage your practice.

While debt financing is usually arranged through an institutional lender, loan arrangements can also be made with a private individual, often a family member. The obvious difficulty is knowing of the existence of those individuals and approaching them in a businesslike manner. While your approach to borrowing from private lenders like friends or family members may be more relaxed, those situations still require proper legal documentation and appropriate independent advice to all parties.

PRACTICE POINT

It is easier to secure a loan from an institutional lender if you understand the lender's desire to document the transaction and obtain adequate security and collateral. Often you will feel that an institutional lender is over-secured; if this is the case, attempt to negotiate the release of certain security from the lender's requirements. Remember that you are a valuable customer of the lender. Make sure that the terms of the loan are reasonable and will not deprive you of the flexibility necessary in your practice.

LOAN ARRANGEMENTS

DIRECT LOANS

The form of loan your practice obtains will depend, among other things, on your creditworthiness — your billing forecasts, your credibility in the community, your years of experience, and your credit history. Once the lender has determined that you are creditworthy, you will be expected to sign certain legal documents setting out the terms of the loan and any secured assets.

The most common bank document used to secure a direct loan is a promissory note, which normally is printed on a standard bank form in the principal amount of the loan. A typical bank promissory note is reproduced in appendix L.

TERM

Usually a business promissory note is payable on demand. You should make sure that other documentation is available, in the form of either a loan agreement or a "comfort letter," that adequately confirms the repayment terms in the event that other terms have been discussed orally and are not incorporated into the written agreement. That other document will specify your obligation to make regular monthly payments of interest or a blended payment of interest and principal, together with the conditions that will bring the loan into default.

As well, the customer should determine whether or not a term loan requires a specified payment at specific times (in which case the bank cannot require a faster repayment) or whether the loan is repayable on a demand basis, even though informal arrangements for repayment have been made.

INTEREST RATES

The interest rate on a business loan can be either fixed or variable. Most business loans are made at a variable rate of interest, based on the prime rate plus a certain percentage. Remember that a variable interest rate loan can create severe financial hardship when interest rates are high or rising.

BLANK NOTES

Often a bank will make a revolving loan in which deposits made by the customer are applied to reduce the amount of the loan outstanding. Further advances are then made, up to an agreed-upon maximum amount outstanding, as funds are needed. In this arrangement, the customer usually provides the bank with a series of signed, but otherwise blank, promissory notes on the understanding that the bank will complete the notes by filling in the principal amount as advances are obtained by the customer, together with the applicable interest.

While this practice is often discouraged, the customer can take some comfort in knowing that banks have a fiduciary duty to their customers to act in good faith. The prudent banker would not attempt to complete such a note unless the proper circumstances warranted such action, having regard to its fiduciary duties to its customers.

DEBENTURES

The debenture, another means of evidence of indebtedness, is typically used only by corporations. A debenture is a form of debt obligation issued by the borrower under which principal and interest are to be paid in accordance with the terms of the document. The debenture may, but need not be, secured by a charge on the assets of the practice or the holding corporation.

MAKING THE LOAN

When a loan is granted, you will normally be asked to sign a formal agreement with the lending institution. Generally speaking, the agreement will be either a commitment letter or a loan agreement.

COMMITMENT LETTER

A typical commitment letter confirms that a bank is willing to grant a loan to your practice on certain terms. Upon acceptance by you, the commitment letter constitutes your agreement to obtain funding and repay the loan on the basis of the terms set out in the letter. Among other things, the commitment letter will indicate whether the amounts are repayable on demand or in accordance with a fixed repayment schedule, specify the interest rate, record and describe any secured assets, and describe the conditions in which the loan will be brought into default.

LOAN AGREEMENT

A loan agreement is, in essence, a contract with respect to debt financing. The loan agreement is often used in cases where substantial debt is incurred over a long period, and includes covenants relating to the reporting of the financial position of the practice, debt-equity ratios to be maintained, and a strict definition of events that will bring the loan into default. In addition, there may be positive covenants from the bank with respect to the "working out" of a severe default in the loan agreement in accordance with various terms. Typically, a loan agreement will also contain "negative covenants" from the borrower, confirming that he or she will not undertake certain business activities, such as the acquisition of new equipment, without the consent of the bank.

INSTITUTIONAL SECURITY

Too often veterinarians fail to approach an institutional lender confidently enough because they feel that they are not in a position to provide enough security or collateral to obtain a loan. In this section we will discuss the types of security and collateral that institutional lenders are likely to accept, so that you may analyse your creditworthiness and prepare an adequate loan application.

By taking collateral, the bank ensures that the assets that are pledged as security may be used to satisfy all or a portion of the debt owed. Two types of loans are commonly provided by most institutional lenders: an operating loan (usually granted to finance inventories and receivables) and a term loan (granted to finance the purchase of tangible assets used in the practice). You should have those uses in mind when you approach the bank.

GENERAL ASSIGNMENT OF RECEIVABLES

One of the most popular forms of security requested by banks is an assignment of debts owed to the practice through accounts receivable. Often, a standard form of agreement is used, which permits the bank to notify your clients to pay their accounts directly to the bank. Most banks will not take this action unless you have defaulted on your loan repayments, or unless the bank believes that its position has been compromised somehow.

The assignment of receivables provides that all receivables are to be held in trust by the practice for the benefit of the bank. This means that a type of trust relationship is formed between the customer and the bank which previously may not have existed.

As well as a general assignment of accounts receivable, there may be a specific assignment in the event that a clearly defined account is to be used as collateral — such as the receivables of your largest dairy farmer client for which herd management services are provided on a regular basis.

The wording of most general assignments is very general and gives the bank wide powers to include not only accounts receivable but other "book debts," including cash, claims, moneys, and other debts.

This form of security may be registered by the bank pursuant to the provisions of any personal property registration system in the province, and renewed upon expiry.

GENERAL SECURITY AGREEMENT

A security agreement creates a security interest in favour of the lender in certain property of the borrower. In most cases the interest attaches to all the borrower's assets both present and future, and provides specific remedies to the lender in the event that the borrower defaults in the loan arrangement. Among other things, the lender may seize the assets pledged in the general security agreement and appoint a receiver for the practice.

PRACTICE POINT

A general security agreement will usually require that the equipment covered by the agreement be adequately insured against loss during the term of the loan. In addition, there may be restrictions on your ability to sell the collateral other than in the ordinary course of the practice. Be sure that you read the document in its entirety in order to avoid an unintentional breach of the agreement.

It is important for the customer to ensure that the security given to the bank is properly reflected in the general security agreement, and that no other assets are affected. As well, the representations and warranties contained in the agreement with respect to encumbrances on the assets should be reviewed to ensure that they reflect the reality of the situation. Often the bank will demand priority over any other secured creditor.

The general security agreement is normally registered under the personal property registration system in each province. A form of this type of agreement is set out in appendix M.

CHATTEL MORTGAGE

Many banks still employ a document referred to as a "chattel mortgage" to provide a specific security interest in a specified piece of equipment used in the practice. A chattel mortgage is similar to the general security agreement described above; however, it is often restricted to the present assets of the business. For instance, an expensive portable X-ray machine used in a equine practice may be good collateral for the bank.

DEBENTURE

If the borrower is a corporation, such as a veterinary holding corporation, the lender may require a debenture. A debenture is a promise to pay made by the corporation and a mortgage over certain property as security for the repayment of the debt.

Unlike a general security agreement, a debenture can take a "fixed" charge on specific assets, or a "floating" charge on all assets. In the event of default, the floating charge "crystallizes" and all assets subject to the floating charge are then secured by the bank as of that date. Land can be included in the debenture; if it is included, the debenture will be registered in the land registry or land titles office.

Like the general security agreement, the debenture provides various remedies for the lender, which can realize on the security, take possession of it, appoint a receiver, and sell the assets.

LAND MORTGAGE

Most lenders will accept a collateral land mortgage or charge as security for a business purpose. The mortgage sets out the principal and interest repayment terms and provides security on the lands owned by the business.

As in other real estate transactions, the bank will require a legal opinion that the borrower has good and marketable title to the property. This means that your solicitor will have to search the title of the land described in the mortgage. A collateral mortgage does not necessarily have to be given for the land and buildings from which your practice is carried on; you may pledge an interest in your personal residence or cottage property.

PRACTICE POINT

A land mortgage contains very effective remedies for the mortgagee that can be implemented quickly to remedy default in the mortgage. The relative cost of placing this type of security is high in comparison with other forms. For these reasons, a land mortgage should not be used for securing a loan; however, if a large loan is required, a land mortgage may be inevitable.

GUARANTEE

A personal guarantee from the partners of a practice and, in some cases, their spouses is often the security of choice of many lenders. The guarantee can be unlimited, or limited to a specific amount. In the case of a spousal guarantee, the bank will often require that the non-owning spouse seek independent legal advice before signing the guarantee.

A guarantee often contains an assignment and postponement of claims on the profits of the practice in favour of the bank. Thus, if a partner is owed money from the practice, his or her repayment is postponed in favour of the lender, who has priority as to repayment.

Too often the acute need for funding blurs the borrower's vision. Business financing is a competitive field; chartered banks, trust companies, and other lenders are eager to attract new customers. It is incumbent upon the borrower to seek out and maintain a relationship with a lender that is interested in your future growth, and that acts in a reasonable manner with respect to your security arrangements.

BASIC TAX PLANNING

The implications of taxation law are far-reaching, and have a direct influence on the success of your practice. Figuratively speaking, Revenue Canada is a silent partner in your clinic, and deserves great respect. The astute practitioner will be familiar with basic taxation concepts and strategies in order to take maximum advantage of the tax rules.

PRACTICE POINT

Effective tax planning is key to effective practice management. In many respects Revenue Canada is a silent partner in your practice. The effect of tax law is pervasive, and a basic knowledge of taxation is required.

In this chapter we will discuss some of those concepts in an effort to provide you with a greater understanding of this complex legislation. A familiarity with this topic can only assist you in making your clinic as successful and profitable as possible.

WHO IS TAXED?

Different countries employ different criteria to determine which persons are subject to the payment of tax to their government: citizenship, domicile, residence, and geographic location. In Canada, the criterion for tax liability is "residence." Every "person" who is "resident" in Canada at any time of the year is potentially liable for the payment of income tax.

A "person" can be either an individual or a corporation. An individual is resident in Canada if he or she has "sojourned" in Canada for at least 183 days in the year. A corporation is deemed to be a resident of Canada if it was incorporated in Canada after April 26, 1965. For a veterinary practice, this criterion would relate to income earned by a holding corporation or by the operating corporation in provinces where incorporation of a practice is permitted. In addition, a corporation is deemed to be a resident if the "central management and control" is in Canada, on the basis of a number of tests, including the location of the registered office, the principal place of business, and the residence of the directors.

Canada is a signatory to many international tax treaties. The provisions of those treaties determine, among other things, whether income tax is payable to either of the countries that are parties to the treaty.

INCOME FOR TAX PURPOSES

The federal Income Tax Act (ITA) provides for the payment to the federal government of a levy based on income. The federal government collects the tax and remits a portion to the provincial government. Income tax is payable on net income — that is, income after all applicable deductions and tax credits have been calculated.

INCOME FROM EMPLOYMENT

The ITA describes in great detail what is to be included in income from employment. Of primary importance, especially in connection with the deductibility of expenses, is the determination whether one is an employee or self-employed as an independent contractor (see chapter 5). Essentially, an employee renders service, while a self-employed person provides services. An employee acts under the control and direction of his or her employer.

Obviously, the earnings of the employed veterinarian are to be included in the determination of income for tax purposes. Other types of income must also be included — for example, employee benefits received in the tax year by virtue of the employment. Such things as pension contributions, group sickness and disability plan payments on behalf of the employee, and deferred profit-sharing plan contributions must be included in the calculation of gross income.

PRACTICE POINT

Many veterinarians will start out as employees of a practice. Income tax will be deducted at source from your regular paycheque. You will be issued a T4 slip by your employer, which records the amount and type of deductions made. You are required to file a tax return for the year no later than April 30 in the following year.

INCOME FROM BUSINESS

Section 9 of the ITA provides that a taxpayer's income for the year must include profit from a business carried on by the taxpayer. Other provisions set out specific types of profits to be included: income from services performed in the tax year, bad debts recovered, and royalties. The veterinarian who owns a practice will have this type of business income.

INCOME FROM PROPERTY

The ITA states that income derived from any property owned by the taxpayer must be included in income. Rents received from real estate investments, dividends received from shareholdings, and loan interest received must be included.

INCOME VERSUS CAPITAL

Before we look at the allowable deductions from gross income, it is important to note the distinction made in the ITA between "income" and "capital." Because these sources of revenue are treated differently, the taxpayer must be able to recognize whether a particular receipt is of an income or a capital nature.

There is a great deal of case law relating to the difference between income and capital. Generally, the courts have used the "fruit and the tree" analogy to make their decisions; that is, capital is the "tree" and any investment income derived therefrom is the "fruit." Thus, the "fruit" is treated as income, while the disposition of the "tree" that gives rise to revenue is treated as capital. Other tests are used by the courts in making the determination, such as the subject matter of the property, the length of ownership, the frequency of similar transactions by the same taxpayer, improvements to the property, and the taxpayer's motive.

PRACTICE POINT

Some of the most significant tax policies developed in recent years relate to the treatment of capital gains. At present, capital gains are given preferential treatment over income; you should attempt to plan carefully for the disposition of capital property so as to achieve the greatest tax advantage.

The most important outcome of the distinction between income and capital has to do with the capital gains rules, which are discussed below.

DEDUCTIONS

As previously mentioned, the ITA imposes tax liability only on net income. The act provides for a number of statutory deductions from gross income to be used in arriving at the taxable income figure.

DEDUCTIONS FROM EMPLOYMENT INCOME

The ITA contains a detailed list of those expenses that may be deducted from employment income. Generally, the employee is granted a "blanket" deduction for employment expenses — either a fixed amount or a percentage of income.

In addition to the "blanket" deduction, a number of specific deductions are permitted; however, the ability to benefit from those deductions depends largely on one's type of employment: legal expenses for the collection of a salary or wage, expenses incurred for the purpose of earning income (available to commissioned salespeople), or professional dues payments (such as annual fees for membership in a provincial veterinary regulatory body). These are only a few of the deductions that are available in addition to the other general deductions for such things as alimony payments, child care expenses, RRSPs, and tuition fees.

DEDUCTIONS FROM BUSINESS AND PROPERTY INCOME

PRACTICE POINT

Keep accurate records and receipts for deductible expenses. In the event of an audit, you may be required to present such receipts.

The ITA provides for certain deductions from business and property income. Of greatest importance to the owner of a veterinary practice is the availability for deduction of expenses incurred for the purpose of gaining income. This general rule permits the deduction from income of all expenses of the practice so long as the expenditures were made with a view to making a profit. A veterinarian may properly deduct from business income all or a part of entertainment expenses, automobile expenses, office expenses, wages of employees, and similar items. It is imperative that the taxpayer be able to provide evidence, in the form of receipts, to Revenue Canada in order to defend any assertion that the expense was not made for the purpose of gaining profit.

In addition to the general deductibility rule set out above, a number of statutory deductions are permitted: the capital cost allowance (discussed below), interest, bad debts, an employer's contributions to employee savings plans, certain professional fees, convention fees, and foreign taxes paid.

CAPITAL COST ALLOWANCE

One of the most misunderstood concepts in the income tax legislation is that of the deductibility of capital costs. In essence, the taxpayer is permitted to deduct each year an amount for depreciation on capital property.

The ITA places various types of capital properties into several classes and fixes a specific rate, expressed as a percentage of value, at which that type of property depreciates. The taxpayer is permitted a deduction equal to the undepreciated value of the capital asset times the rate of depreciation. The legislation provides such a deduction on a declining balance basis; that is, the reduced value for one year becomes the base value for the subsequent year to which the percentage deduction is applied.

In the event that the capital property is disposed of for an amount in excess of its undepreciated capital cost, the taxpayer must include the difference as income through a process called "recapture." The taxpayer is permitted a further deduction in the event that the disposition takes place at a value less than the undepreciated capital cost (a "terminal loss"), provided that the capital asset disposed of is not replaced.

The ITA also permits deductions for eligible capital properties, including trademarks, patents, client and patient lists, and other items generally relating to the goodwill of the clinic.

CAPITAL GAINS

The taxation of capital gains is of relatively recent vintage; the provisions were introduced in 1972. This area of income tax legislation has received a great deal of attention in recent years.

A capital gain or capital loss represents the appreciation or loss, respectively, of a capital property not subject to capital cost allowance. A portion of the capital gain — that is, the difference between the "proceeds of disposition" and the "adjusted cost base" — is included in income and taxed at the normal personal or corporate tax rates. In its most simple terms, the quantum of the capital gain or loss is determined by taking the difference between the price you sell the asset for and the costs you incurred when you first acquired it. Likewise, a portion of a capital loss may be deducted against other capital gains. In addition, certain capital losses may be carried forward to other tax years or carried back to previous years.

A capital gain or loss is realized only on the disposition of the capital asset. The most usual case is the sale of an asset to a third party; however, the ITA deems a disposition of the asset to take place upon the death of a taxpayer or upon the taxpayer's leaving the country. This deemed disposition makes it important that you give thoughtful consideration to estate planning issues (discussed in chapter 12).

There are many complex rules governing the computation of a capital gain or loss and the determination of proceeds of disposition. The adjusted cost base of the asset is subject to further rules, which provide for certain amounts to be added to or deducted from the cost base.

Certain types of properties that otherwise would give rise to a capital gain are exempt from the payment of tax. The most common example is the sale of a principal residence.

The most recent change to capital gains taxation relates to the exemption of taxable capital gains, formerly up to $100,000 in one's lifetime. The February 1994 federal budget has abolished this exemption; but taxpayers are permitted to establish a new adjusted cost base for a capital property by making an election in their 1994 tax returns. It is important to note that this exemption is not available to corporations and that special rules apply to certain types of farming properties and small business corporations.

Clearly, capital gains are afforded beneficial tax treatment, and the astute practitioner will take advantage of those benefits whenever possible.

CORPORATE TAX

Although they are persons for tax purposes, corporations are taxed differently from individuals. This is an important concept for veterinary practitioners who have formed a holding corporation to insulate assets from debts of the practice or to maximize tax benefits, and for those who are permitted to incorporate their practices. Generally speaking, the computation of income is similar for both; however, the rates of tax payable on net income differ. Individuals pay tax at three gradually increasing rates of tax, depending on the income received. Corporations are taxed at a fixed combined provincial and federal tax rate, which varies between provinces. In Ontario, the present rate is approximately 50 percent of net income.

Corporate tax rates are initially higher than personal rates; however, depending on the type of corporation being taxed, further deductions are available. For instance, a Canadian-controlled private corporation is entitled to the small business deduction, which reduces the Ontario tax rate to approximately 25 percent of net income. As well, special resource-based or manufacturing corporations are entitled to lower rates of tax.

Profits of a corporation are often distributed by way of a dividend payable on the shares held by the shareholders. The amount of the dividend is then included in the shareholder's income from property in his or her personal tax return.

TAX ADMINISTRATION

The ITA establishes a statutory framework for the administration of the legislation. The act requires that taxpayers, in most cases, must file a tax return annually to report their income. Corporations must file a return for every fiscal year, and individuals must file whenever there is tax payable. A corporation must file within six months of its year-end and an individual must file no later than April 30 in each year.

Upon receipt of the completed return, Revenue Canada must provide an assessment of the tax payable, together with any interest or penalties. In the event that the taxpayer disagrees with the assessment, he or she may file a notice of objection within ninety days from the date of mailing of the notice of assessment. That time limit is strictly enforced; however, the taxpayer may apply to the Tax Court of Canada for an extension of time to file the notice. A hearing may be necessary, together with appeals to the courts.

In addition, the ITA provides for the collection of tax by Revenue Canada, including the issuance of a third-party demand for payment, which requires a third party, such as a bank, to pay funds to Revenue Canada that otherwise would be payable to the taxpayer.

PRACTICE POINT

Self-employed veterinarians usually remit tax quarterly to Revenue Canada. The failure to make the quarterly instalments on the fifteenth day of March, June, September, and December results in interest being charged by Revenue Canada on the amount unpaid. In any event, the total tax to be paid must be remitted with your return not later than April 30 in each year in order to avoid interest and penalties.

Finally, the legislation provides for a number of tax-related offences, including failure to file a return, tax evasion, and failure to keep adequate accounting records.

Income tax legislation in Canada is complex and difficult. It is important that you understand the general principles of taxation and recognize those situations requiring professional assistance.

ACCOUNTS RECEIVABLE MANAGEMENT

Apart from your efforts to promote and provide expert veterinary services, effective control of debts owed to you will lead to greater success in your practice. A clinic with impressive billings can easily run into economic ruin if payments aren't collected. Your ability to identify a problem account and take corrective steps quickly will certainly be reflected in your annual financial statements.

The veterinary legislation in Newfoundland and Labrador gives veterinarians the authority to demand, receive, and sue for in a court "reasonable fees for professional services rendered" and the costs of drugs, antibiotics, and other materials used in those services. The same provision permits the practitioner to be engaged by the province and collect appropriate fees, salaries, or other remuneration.

AVOIDING THE PROBLEM

The simplest means of recovering accounts receivable is to take active steps to avoid the process entirely by keeping debt collection procedures current, but many animal hospitals fail to use the tools available to assist them. A fear of losing a client or a desire to impress a new one often motivates the practitioner to take risks that, in retrospect, were unnecessary. Therefore, it is important to take advantage of the simple and effective procedures for managing your accounts receivable.

DEPOSITS

The simplest means of lessening the negative impact of an account receivable is to require a deposit for the veterinary services you are about to perform. Historically, a deposit was presented to a vendor as an indication of the purchaser's good faith and intention to complete a transaction. The vendor knew that the purchaser was prepared to provide funds in exchange for the vendor's promise to deliver certain goods at a future time.

PRACTICE POINT

Most clients understand the need for paying a deposit, particularly if an expensive surgical procedure is required for an animal. The best time to obtain the deposit is during your first consultation with the client.

In legal terms, a deposit is forfeited by the client in the event that a transaction fails as a result of the client's actions; in other words, you are entitled to keep the deposit if the client fails to pay the balance of the account or otherwise fails to maintain the relationship. For instance, if you had indicated that a follow-up examination was necessary and the client failed to keep the appointment and the animal is not presented again, then the deposit may be kept in satisfaction of the fee for the missed appointment. A good practice management technique would be to post prominent signs stating that fees will be charged for missed appointments.

Obtaining a deposit will not necessarily avoid the accrual of an account receivable; however, it will serve to lessen the sting of an unpaid bill. Most practitioners and office administrators would agree that collecting a portion of the account is better than collecting none of it. The amount of the deposit will vary with the complexity and expense of the procedure to be performed.

The best time to obtain the deposit is in the discussions that precede your engagement for a specific procedure. A simple form of deposit agreement can be included in your consent-to-treatment form when it is reviewed and signed by the client.

SECURED TRANSACTIONS

There are several means by which a veterinarian may obtain tangible security for the payment for his or her professional services. Such security can be enforced relatively quickly in the event that the client fails to pay the account on a timely basis. Another reason for obtaining security relates to the scheme of distribution to creditors in bankruptcy. Should the client make an assignment in bankruptcy, preference will be given to secured creditors. In fact, secured creditors may realize on their security and not be involved in the bankruptcy proceedings at all. You should be aware that a bank or other lender may have priority to the security and that your position may be subject to the rights of the prior lien holder. A typical security agreement is reproduced in appendix M.

Several types of security are available to the clinic and are discussed below.

PERSONAL PROPERTY SECURITY LEGISLATION

The Ontario Personal Property Security Act (PPSA) came into effect in 1976. The PPSA is the most common means of providing for and giving public notice of a security interest in personal property. Similar legislative schemes are found in the Personal Property Security Act of Manitoba and chattel security registration regimes in other provinces. Unlike the registration system, which is used to give notice of interests in land, no central registry for personal property interests is available in most provinces; however, the PPSA and similar acts are quickly moving to fulfil that function.

PRACTICE POINT

The placement of a personal property security is relatively easy and inexpensive. For large-animal practices, the taking of security in the form of collateral in farm equipment or machinery is an effective way of avoiding bad debts.

The legislation sets up uniform methods of creating a security interest between a creditor veterinarian and a debtor client, and deals in types of collateral — consumer goods, inventory, equipment, accounts receivable, and "goods." It is interesting to note that the definition of "goods" in the Ontario legislation specifically includes animals and the unborn young of animals. The creative practitioner in a large-animal practice could potentially claim a security interest in a herd of dairy cattle he or she has treated if the farmer client's account goes into default. Likewise, the farmer could pledge an item of farm equipment to the veterinarian in order to secure the payment of the professional account.

In the event that you wish to obtain security for a portion of an unpaid account, a form of legal contract referred to as a security agreement may be easily entered into and registered. The contracts are often referred to as "general security agreements" or "chattel mortgages" and are in daily use by banks and other financial institutions to secure the repayment of a loan. Registration gives public notice of your prior claim to any person who may wish to acquire an interest in the same property. As well, it sets up a system of priorities for payment among persons claiming an interest in the same collateral.

Similarly, the context of a small-animal practice, the veterinarian may wish to obtain a security interest in the proceeds of the sale of puppies delivered by caesarean section by you for the benefit of the kennel owner.

The most important aspect of the PPSA relates to the enforcement of a debt and the remedy sections that can be used if the debt goes into default. In addition to commencing a court action against the debtor for payment, the secured party is permitted to obtain possession of the goods, appoint a receiver, and retain and dispose of the collateral; these procedures are similar to power of sale proceedings in a land mortgage. The remedies may be very important if the value of the particular good is vulnerable to speedy depreciation. For example, the large-animal practitioner who possesses a security interest on a tractor could later seize and sell the tractor to satisfy his account. This may seem like an extraordinary action; however, if you value the special skills you have developed in the medical assistance to the herd, then you should likewise value getting paid for those services, which have, in effect, permitted the farmer to earn an income.

REAL ESTATE MORTGAGES

On rare occasions, especially if complex surgery is to be performed on large animals, a special type of account may be in order. Depending on the amount of that account, it may be necessary to obtain a mortgage on real estate owned by the client. Typically, the client would sign a promissory note that sets out a repayment schedule. The note would then be collaterally secured by a mortgage on the land, which would be registered in the appropriate land registry office. The costs of the registration would be added to the promissory note in most instances. Should the note go into default, the veterinarian will be at liberty to exercise the very strong remedies of foreclosure and power of sale contained in the mortgage.

REPAIR AND STORAGE LIEN ACT

In October 1989 the Ontario government gave final approval to legislation providing for the registration of a lien on personal property. The Repair and Storage Lien Act (RSLA) has been the subject of much debate in veterinary circles in that province.

The RSLA essentially provides for two forms of liens on personal property — possessory and non-possessory. In the case of a clinic, the property affected would be the animal itself — the patient that has been treated but not yet released to its owner. The RSLA provides that so long as you retain possession of the animal you have a lien on it, and you need not release it until your account is paid. In the event that you have "written evidence of indebtedness," the animal may be released, and your non-possessory lien will continue. Ultimately, if the account remains unpaid, you are permitted, after giving proper notice, to sell the animal and apply the proceeds to your account.

The legislation raises certain difficulties in a veterinary context: first, the value of the animal is often much less than the amount of the overdue account; second, as a result of a decision of the Ontario Health Disciplines Board in 1991, there has been significant debate relating to the professional ethics of using an animal as a "lever" to force the payment of the account. The College of Veterinarians of Ontario has indicated that its previous abandoned animal policy has been superseded by the RSLA, and has noted the practical difficulties associated with its use; that is, the continued care, feeding, exercise, and grooming of the animal and their attendant costs. The college has suggested that it is more likely to be in the veterinarian's best interest to return the animal and sue for outstanding fees. In essence, the RSLA dictates that you need not hold the animal "for ransom" provided that you have a written acknowledgment of indebtedness. The remedy of sale of the animal takes a period of time to implement; thus, any ransom issue is, to a great extent, removed. Ample time is permitted in the RSLA for the client to make satisfactory arrangements to pay your reasonable account. You should be aware that an excessive fee charged by the practitioner could lead to difficulties in the use of this remedy if the failure to pay is based solely on the fact that the fee was unreasonable in the circumstances.

It is mandatory that your account forms be reviewed to ensure that they provide the necessary information, and that an office policy be implemented to ensure that the forms are always signed. A form of acknowledgment that may be added to your present invoice format (appendix N) is reproduced in appendix O.

Section 36 of the Saskatchewan Veterinarians Act states that a member of the Saskatchewan Veterinary Medical Association has a lien on any animal in his or her possession for the price of food, care, attendance, accommodation, treatment, medicine, or professional services furnished by the veterinarian. This lien is in addition to any other remedy available to the practitioner and permits the veterinarian to "detain in his custody and sell, subject to this section, the animal of any person who is indebted to him for feeding, sheltering, housing, confining, boarding, treating or caring for an animal." Such a lien has priority over any other interest in the animal. So long as the practitioner adequately provides for the animal while it is in his or her possession, then, if the animal is not reclaimed within thirty days, the veterinarian is authorized to sell the animal to reclaim the costs with respect to the lien and the detention. Obviously, where a sale is intended, notice of the sale must be given to the animal's owner, and the practitioner must account for the sale proceeds to the owner. The proceeds will be applied first to the expenses associated with the sale itself, and second to the debt that gave rise to the lien. In the event that the animal is not sold, the veterinarian may destroy or otherwise dispose of the animal.

Obviously, resort to this type of remedy involving the sale or destruction of an animal cannot be taken lightly. All possible alternatives should be exhausted prior to implementing this strategy. The real value of these lien remedies is the negotiating value provided to the practitioner. While these solutions are somewhat viable in a large-animal clinic, in a small-animal clinic, given the relative low value of companion animals, it is unlikely that the use of these powers will be truly effective.

What is important about the Saskatchewan lien rights is that they appear only to be available *before* the practitioner loses possession of the animal, in contrast to the Ontario legislation, which provides for a non-possessory lien in certain circumstances. The effectiveness of this remedy probably lies in its "policing" attributes; an owner is more likely to pay the account when he or she knows that the animal might be detained and sold. On the other hand, the usefulness of the remedy should not be overestimated, as the value of the animal will, in most contentious cases, be much less than the account outstanding.

PROOF OF INDEBTEDNESS

It is sometimes difficult to prove that a debt is actually owed. Effective records management is of primary importance, particularly if collection proceedings proceed as far as litigation. An invoice signed by the client is a bare minimum. Depending on the amount of the debt and the client's creditworthiness, you may wish to have the client execute a promissory note, which provides very good evidence of indebtedness. A promissory note does not act as security; however, properly drafted, it shows that the debtor is aware of the debts outstanding.

QUANTUM MERUIT

In collecting your accounts for professional services, you should be aware of a legal principle known as "quantum meruit" (literally, "as much as he deserves"). Sometimes practitioners fail to discuss fully with the client the manner, extent, and cost of treatments before rendering the service. Later, after the treatment has been performed, the client feels that the bill is too high and refuses to pay on the basis that no contract existed because the fundamental terms of the contract for service, such as the fee to be charged, were not agreed upon. Fortunately, the doctrine of quantum meruit applies in these cases. That doctrine holds that, notwithstanding the fact that no contract may have existed, the practitioner is entitled in equity to be paid a fair fee for his or her services. In *Marquis Road Veterinary Medical Centre Ltd. v. Goebel* ((1985), 39 Sask. R. 170) facts similar to the situation described above were presented to the Saskatchewan Provincial Court. The judge found that the veterinarian was entitled to compensation on the basis of quantum meruit and awarded the veterinarian a judgment of $160.

Similarly, in *Schmidt v. Equine Veterinary Centre* (25 ACWS (2d) 181), a 1983 decision of the British Columbia County Court, the veterinary clinic was found to be entitled to payment for services performed, notwithstanding that the attending veterinarian did not receive instructions to proceed with the services from the correct person. The practitioner responded to an emergency call from an employee at a stable and determined that a horse was gravely ill. The horse was euthanized after the veterinarian had obtained a second opinion. The owner of the horse refused to pay the veterinary bill. The court held that the veterinarian reasonably believed that he acted upon authorized instructions from the owner's agent, and that the owner was responsible for payment.

DEMAND FOR PAYMENT

At common law, in most provinces, a demand for payment must be made before any collection remedies are used. The amount of notice required varies with the circumstances — the amount of the debt, the risk of loss or damage, and the prospect of an animal being taken out of the jurisdiction. A typical form of demand for payment is set out in appendix P.

The regulations under the Professional Code and Veterinary Surgeons Act of Quebec are an interesting departure from the statutes of the other provinces. In the event that a client disputes the professional fee, the client must, before seeking arbitration, apply to a syndic, or investigator, for conciliation. If the dispute is not resolved by the syndic, the client may submit the issue to arbitration as set out in the legislation.

The Veterinary Medical Act of Manitoba provides that a veterinarian in that province is "entitled to demand from a person by whom he is consulted or employed, and to recover in court, reasonable charges for professional services rendered for or on behalf of that person and the cost of medicines or medical appliances supplied by the member in his [or her] professional capacity."

In the Northwest Territories, no person is entitled to receive a professional fee in the practice of veterinary surgery unless he or she holds a licence under the Veterinary Profession Act in that jurisdiction.

THE COURT SYSTEM

It is important to understand the court structure in your province and be familiar with the litigation process so that you can make an informed decision whether to bring an action against a client for the collection of a debt.

SMALL CLAIMS COURT

The Provincial Court (Civil Division), or the Small Claims Court, as it is more commonly known in most provinces, is a simple but usually effective means of debt collection. In a relatively informal setting, the parties to a dispute appear before a judge. Often, neither party will engage a lawyer; rather, the preparation of court documents and appearances in court are usually undertaken by the opposing litigants.

In Ontario, the Small Claims Court has jurisdiction in any action where the amount claimed does not exceed $6,000. A claim for a larger amount must be brought either in one of the other courts or lowered to fall within the jurisdiction of the Small Claims Court. Other provinces have different monetary thresholds: in British Columbia the limit is $10,000; in Prince Edward Island and Newfoundland the limit is $3,000.

Court proceedings are commenced by the issuance of a statement of claim, which asserts that a debt is owing for the sale of a good or the provision of services. Claim forms may be obtained from the local Small Claims Court and deposited with the court clerk to be served on the defendant. The defendant is then permitted a short period in which to file a statement of dispute, if any.

Once a statement of dispute has been received by the clerk, or the time for delivering the statement has expired, the clerk will provide the parties with a notice of trial or a notice of default judgment.

Notwithstanding that the Small Claims Court is less formal than the higher courts, the same principles of law apply. You must show adequate evidence of the amount owing to you and the reasons why the debt arose in the first place, together with evidence of your efforts to collect the debt.

HIGHER COURTS

In Ontario, the Ontario Court (General Division) has jurisdiction to hear cases involving claims above $6,000. In Alberta, the equivalent court is the Court of Queen's Bench. These courts are presided over by a judge. As in the Small Claims Court, actions are commenced by the issuance of a statement of claim, which is served upon the debtor. The debtor then has an opportunity to file a statement of defence.

PRACTICE POINT

The court process, at any level, can be time-consuming and expensive, as well as emotionally stressful. Effective practice management should be directed at avoiding the court process and, if litigation is unavoidable, streamlining the process and presenting persuasive evidence.

You may appear personally in the higher courts, although solicitors normally act for the parties to actions at this level. The process is formal, and there are a great number of complicated rules of practice that must be followed in order to continue the proceeding. The rules also involve time limitations which, if not met, may seriously compromise your case.

COURT PROCEEDINGS

When you bring an action in a higher court, your solicitor may use legal terminology that you find confusing. In this section of the chapter, we will discuss the court process so that you can better understand the actions of your lawyer. The examples set out are based on the Ontario law; similar provisions exist in the other provinces.

PLEADINGS

As mentioned above, a court action is commenced by the issuance of a statement of claim similar to that which appears in appendix Q. The statement of claim sets out the facts which you, the plaintiff, are alleging. The drafting of pleadings is subject to many rules, and is best left to the experienced solicitor. The statement of claim is issued by the court staff upon payment of a fee. In contrast to Small Claims Court, it is up to the plaintiff to have the statement of claim served on the defendant. In most cases, service must be made personally — that is, the defendant must accept the document in person.

Once the statement of claim has been served, the defendant has a period of time, usually twenty days, within which to file a statement of defence. Failure to do so will result in a default judgment in favour of the plaintiff. The statement of defence usually alleges a breach of contract by the plaintiff, such as a discrepancy in the fee agreed to or a failure to perform services in the manner the defendant required.

When the pleadings have been exchanged, each of the parties will have an understanding of the issues that will eventually be argued in court.

DEFAULT JUDGMENT

If the defendant fails to deliver a statement of defence within a specified time, the plaintiff may ask the court registrar to enter a default judgment against him or her immediately. It is important to understand, however, that a default judgment can be obtained in this summary fashion only if there is a clear and defined debt outstanding, as set out in the statement of claim. It is not unusual to obtain judgment in debt collection proceedings, because there is typically no justification for the defendant's failure to pay the account. Nonetheless, the plaintiff suffers aggravation and incurs legal expenses in order to obtain that judgment.

THE DISCOVERY PROCESS

Once the action has been commenced and a defence has been offered, the parties to the dispute exchange detailed information about the contents of the pleadings. This process is called "discovery." The rules of practice provide for various means of discovery. The process provides each party with information upon which to base a decision to proceed to a trial, abandon the litigation, or seek a negotiated settlement.

The discovery process is conducted by way of an oral examination or deposition and the presentation of written documentation that will be relied upon during the course of the trial.

COSTS

One of the most widely misunderstood aspects of the debt collection process relates to the awarding of court costs to the successful party in litigation. Our system does not provide for the reimbursement of all expenses and costs incurred by the successful party, whether it be the plaintiff or defendant, in any court proceeding; only a partial reimbursement is available.

The costs of litigation can be significant, especially if one proceeds to trial; accordingly, the cost factor becomes an important element in determining a strategy for the collection of a debt. As will be discussed later, obtaining a successful judgment does not necessarily mean that you will receive full payment. Lawsuits should not be commenced solely for reasons of principle: the prudent plaintiff must also consider the cost of proceeding with the action, along with the risks associated with an unsuccessful lawsuit, in the light of the amount owed.

ENFORCING THE JUDGMENT

The next step in the litigation process relates to enforcing the judgment handed down by the court. Several enforcement mechanisms are available.

PRACTICE POINT

The process after obtaining judgment in your favour is just as important as the legal steps taken to receive the judgment. You must be diligent in your collection proceedings to ensure that effective post-judgment attempts have been made to ensure payment of your account.

EXAMINATION OF THE DEBTOR

The rules of court provide that an unsuccessful defendant may be subjected to an oral examination to determine the extent and whereabouts of his or her assets. Unless the creditor is fully familiar with the debtor's assets, an examination of this nature should be held in order to determine the location and assess the relative value of any assets to be seized and sold to satisfy the judgment. A debtor's failure to attend at an examination can result in imprisonment for contempt of court.

WRIT OF SEIZURE AND SALE

The most popular method of enforcing a judgment is through the filing of a writ of seizure and sale, sometimes referred to as an execution, against the judgment debtor. Provincial legislation provides that once judgment has been obtained, the successful party may, for a small fee, file an execution with the sheriff in every court jurisdiction where the debtor may have assets. The effect of the execution is to charge or encumber all of the debtor's assets in that jurisdiction to the extent of the judgment amount and any interest that accrues thereon. As well, the judgment creditor may instruct the sheriff to seize and sell the debtor's assets to satisfy the debt once the location and value of those assets have been determined.

Sometimes it may take years for a judgment debt to be enforced; for example, the debtor may eventually attempt to sell land against which an execution is filed. It is important to remember that interest accrues on the judgment from the date it is obtained, and is recoverable through the execution.

GARNISHMENT

Garnishment is another remedy available to a person who has successfully obtained a judgment against a debtor. Once a judgment has been obtained, the successful creditor may give a notice to any person (most commonly an employer) who owes money to the judgment debtor. A portion of the money (such as wages) payable to the debtor is then paid directly to the judgment creditor in satisfaction of the judgment. Once again, failure to comply with a garnishment order by an employer may result in contempt-of-court proceedings. Note that under some provincial laws a certain percentage of wages to be received by a debtor will be exempt from garnishment.

It is important to ensure that you receive fair payment for your professional services. In some instances it may be necessary to resort to the legal system to collect debts. Your familiarity with the system will lessen any anxiety you might have about the process, and will enable you to instruct your solicitor knowledgeably.

RISK MANAGEMENT

Canadians live in an increasingly litigious society. Citizens are very much aware of their ability to enforce their legal rights whenever they feel they have been wronged. This phenomenon has manifested itself in a plethora of lawsuits against professionals. It is comforting to note that veterinarians, relative to other professionals, have had few actions brought against them. Nonetheless, to avoid lawsuits, and to ensure the profitability of your practice and the absence of anxiety on the part of the professional staff, you should have an effective plan of risk management in place.

PROFESSIONAL NEGLIGENCE

At common law, any person who holds himself or herself out as having a particular skill owes a duty of care to his or her client to exercise that skill properly. The standard of care is one of "reasonableness" — that is, what would the reasonable veterinarian have done or not done if he or she was faced with the situation in question? If your actions fall below that standard of care, you will have acted negligently. Further, there must be clear evidence of causation — that is, your actions must have led directly to the injury complained of. Provided that you have exercised your skills diligently and competently, the likelihood of your facing an action in negligence is lessened if you have also obtained written informed consent to treatment from the animal's owner.

To succeed in an action alleging professional negligence, the complainant must prove that a duty of care was owed, that the duty of care was breached, and that a financial loss was sustained.

In *Southwhite Stables Inc. v. Ingram Veterinary Services Ltd.* (Alberta Court of Queen's Bench, April 19, 1984, unreported), an experienced veterinarian treated a horse for a vision problem. The specific facts of the case, which involved a pre-purchase inspection of the horse and the opinions expressed as a result of the inspection, are less important than the finding of the court. The court held that the standard of care that is to be met by the veterinary practitioner is identical to that which must be met by a physician. It is not enough to say that your normal practice is to do X; X must be the right thing to do. The veterinarian's duty of care is discharged if his or her actions coincide with the actions rightly accepted by a body of skilled and experienced veterinarians.

In *Hihn v. Shaeffer* ((1988), 8 ACWS (3d) 91), an Ontario Small Claims Court action, a veterinarian was found not to have been negligent in failing to diagnose a ruptured triceps tendon in a dog that had fallen off a bed. Evidence showed that such an injury was unusual and difficult to diagnose.

Sometimes the debate over what constitutes an appropriate standard of care can result in a "battle of the experts" in a court proceeding.

INFORMED CONSENT

A veterinarian should never treat an animal without obtaining the consent of the animal's owner. Failure to obtain consent can result in an action in trespass. (In this context, "trespass" means an unlawful interference with someone else's property.) In addition to holding that the person who consents to the animal's treatment is legally capable of granting consent and that the consent is voluntary, the courts have, at least in the context of human medicine, required that consent be *informed*. It is this requirement that causes the greatest difficulty in the day-to-day management of a busy practice. Impatient clients who have endured long waits in the reception room can too often lead to your proceeding with a particular treatment without properly obtaining written informed consent.

PRACTICE POINT

In a busy practice, all professionals and lay staff members should be aware of the need to obtain owners' written informed consent to the treatment of their animals. While the legal obligation to obtain consent rests with the veterinarian, it is important that clinic managers and lay staff ensure that no treatment proceeds until written informed consent is obtained.

The Supreme Court of Canada has held that in obtaining the consent of a human patient to medical treatment, the physician must answer all specific questions posed by the patient as to the risks involved, and should, without being questioned, disclose to the patient the nature of the proposed treatment, its gravity, the probable risks, the material possible risks, and any special or unusual risks attendant on the procedure. Presumably, the veterinarian must disclose similar types of risks to an animal's owner.

Whether or not these issues have been properly addressed is to be determined with reference to the circumstances of each case. In any event, the discussion should be well documented.

Probable risks and material possible risks are discussed in more detail below, under the heading "Extra-Label Drug Use."

A court's determination will be based on whether a reasonable person in the client's position would have consented to the procedure if there had been proper disclosure of the risks. This point is important: note that the test is *not* based on what information a reasonable veterinarian would disclose in the circumstances. Therefore, the prudent practitioner will err on the side of caution: better to provide too much information than too little.

In Quebec, the risks to be addressed are set out in the statutory Code of Ethics for Veterinary Surgeons. The practitioner must reveal to his or her client, in a complete and objective manner, the nature and scope of the problem, which, in the practitioner's opinion, results from the facts presented to him or her. Further, the practitioner must not express his or her opinion on the basis of incomplete advice, having regard to the examinations conducted by the veterinarian and the information provided by the client.

PRACTICE POINT

It is a good idea for the clinic manager to review all patient files periodically so as to ensure that the required consent forms have been properly executed by the patients' owners. In periodic management meetings the staff can report on and remedy any case files that do not contain the appropriate consent forms.

EMERGENCY TREATMENT

Although no Canadian cases have yet addressed the issue of owners' consent to the emergency medical treatment of animals, it appears likely that when emergency treatment is necessary to preserve the life or future health of a patient and it is impossible to obtain the informed consent of the owner, the veterinarian is privileged to proceed with the treatment.

EVIDENCE OF CONSENT

When a veterinarian cannot produce evidence showing that an owner was given full disclosure of risks associated with a treatment, the court will rely solely on the credibility of the witnesses — the bereaved owner and the professional practitioner. To avoid such a situation, make sure that your practice has in place a routine for obtaining and filing consent forms. A typical consent form is reproduced in appendix o.

At a minimum, the consent form should state that the client has been informed of the probable and possible risks associated with the treatment; ideally, it should set out the specific risks that were discussed. Failure to include the specific risks may lead the court to view the form as not credible.

For certain procedures, such as spaying and neutering, a practice may develop a standard form of consent. Staff should be cautioned against relying exclusively on such standard forms; if an animal presents a condition or symptom that would give rise to risks other than those specified on the standard form, those risks must be spelled out.

Standard-form documents issued in contexts other than veterinary medicine have often been overturned by the courts. If your practice makes use of standard consent forms, it is important that its provisions be specifically pointed out to the client, and that the client be advised to read the form before signing it.

In addition, you should be aware that liability may arise if you fail to disclose certain risks because you believe that the owner will not consent to the treatment if they are disclosed. In normal circumstances, no liability will attach to your failure to act if you are *instructed* not to act.

LIMITATION PERIODS

An action in negligence must be brought by the plaintiff within a certain period of time. A failure to initiate proceedings within the time specified by statute or regulation will effectively bar any claim against a defendant. The Veterinary Medical Act of Newfoundland and Labrador provides that an action for negligence or malpractice against a practitioner must be brought within six months of the date on which the event complained of occurred. In New Brunswick, the Veterinarians Act establishes a limitation period of two years in actions for negligence, malpractice, or breach of contract. Manitoba also imposes a two-year limitation period. In Saskatchewan, any action for negligence against a veterinarian must be brought within one year of the event complained of.

DAMAGES

Damages awarded to plaintiffs in successful actions in negligence are often limited to the value of the dead or injured animal. In *Murray v. Mouris et al.* ((1980), 40 NSR (2d) 637), a decision of the Nova Scotia Supreme Court, the defendant veterinarian had advised a farmer that the farmer's expensive heifer could not reproduce. The farmer arranged for the animal's slaughter. In the slaughtering process the animal was discovered to be five months pregnant. The court found the veterinarian negligent in not ascertaining that the animal was pregnant. The damages were set at $10,000 less the value of the carcass. The award included $2,000 in compensation for the loss of the unborn calf.

In a 1989 case, *Ryan v. Avenue Animal Hospital Ltd.* (241 APR 405), unsuccessful cryosurgery was performed on a standardbred horse. In this case the veterinarian admitted negligence, so the only question for the New Brunswick Court of Queen's Bench was the quantum of damages. At the time of surgery, the horse was valued at $16,800, and damages were awarded in that amount. Expert testimony is often required to determine appropriate monetary damages. The burden of proving the value of the animal rests with the plaintiff.

EXTRA-LABEL DRUG USE

Extra-label or off-label drug use, which involves the administration of a drug in a quantity or for a duration not contemplated by the manufacturer, or the treatment of a species with a drug not intended for that species, is currently a topic of much discussion in the profession.

Practitioners who engage in extra-label drug use argue that increased dosages or durations may enhance the efficacy of the drug, and that it is a shortcoming on the part of the regulatory authorities to withhold approval for such uses. Regardless of the merits of this argument, the practitioner should be aware that the extra-label use of drugs is especially risky in companion animals, who are usually small and who may not be able to tolerate higher dosages of a drug. For example, penicillin is often prescribed in dosages higher than those specified on the manufacturer's label to ensure its effectiveness. But what happens if the animal reacts to the drug in a way that was unanticipated, and dies or is injured?

The issue of professional negligence was discussed above, along with the need to obtain informed consent from an animal's owner before any treatment is undertaken. Before we can adequately deal with these matters as they relate to extra-label drug use, it will be helpful to review the legislation that governs the use of drugs in Canada.

The provisions of the Food and Drug Act (FDA) and of the Narcotic Control Act (NCA) regulate the use of all prescription, controlled, and narcotic drugs. The FDA regulates the distribution of prescription drugs throughout the country.

The term "drug" includes any substance or mixture manufactured, sold, or represented for use in the diagnosis, treatment, mitigation, or prevention of a disease, disorder, or abnormal physical state of a human or an animal. This definition is broad enough to include any compound that has a use intended to fall within the definition. For our purposes, the term will be used here to include any substance used in the medical treatment of an animal.

In both the FDA and the NCA the term "practitioner" includes veterinarians as well as physicians and dentists. The term "prescription" refers to any authorization given by a practitioner for the dispensing of a drug named in the legislation or its accompanying schedules or regulations.

The FDA defines "label" to mean any legend, word, or mark attached to, included in, belonging to, or accompanying any food, drug, cosmetic, device, or package. Any use of a drug that is not contemplated in any label, whether or not the label is affixed to the container, constitutes an extra-label use of the drug.

The FDA and the NCA, along with their accompanying regulations, confer a broad authority for a practitioner to issue a prescription for a drug, having regard to its label. The Veterinarians Act of Ontario, and similar legislation in other provinces, imposes certain further restrictions, to be discussed below.

THE PROFESSIONAL STANDARD

In *Hopp v. Lepp* ([1980] 2 SCR 192) and *Reibl v. Hughes* ((1980), 14 CCLT), both of which were decided in the early 1980s and both of which dealt with the medical treatment of human beings, the Supreme Court of Canada said that the standard to be met in obtaining consent requires "full" disclosure, not merely the degree of disclosure that satisfies a "professional standard." This means that a veterinarian cannot argue that he or she disclosed as much information as a reasonably prudent veterinarian would have disclosed in the same circumstances. The duty of care owed to the client is higher: the veterinarian must disclose the amount of information that a *reasonable pet owner would want to know* in similar circumstances. In other words, the veterinarian must put himself or herself in the owner's position.

The cases dictate that the veterinarian must answer all specific questions posed by the owner as to the risks of extra-label drug use and should, without being asked, disclose the nature of the proposed treatment, its gravity, the probable risks, the material possible risks, and any special or unusual risks attendant upon the treatment.

A risk of death or paralysis, no matter how remote a possibility, must be disclosed in every case.

PROBABLE RISKS

The veterinarian is obliged to use his or her professional resources to provide adequate disclosure of the probable risks of extra-label drug use. But, one might ask, if a use is not set out on a label, how can the practitioner have any knowledge of the probable risks? Consultations with other practitioners and a thorough review of the professional literature may offer an answer to that question. In addition, veterinary consultants employed by the drug manufacturer are normally available to provide this type of information. For a listing of contact persons in a number of pharmaceutical houses, see the January 1993 issue of *Focus,* the official publication of the Ontario Veterinary Medical Association.

MATERIAL POSSIBLE RISKS

What constitutes a material possible risk, and thus a risk that must be disclosed, is a question of fact. What the veterinarian knew or ought to have known about the circumstances of the animal and the owner goes to the duty to disclose material risks. For example, the use of a drug that may affect a dog's fertility is of material importance to a breeder, and must be disclosed. If the owner is not a breeder and plans to have the animal spayed or neutered as soon as it is old enough, the risk of infertility is not material.

Whether or not a risk is material may have to be determined on the basis of expert evidence. However, the courts have placed less importance on expert opinion and greater importance on the relationship between the owner and the veterinarian. Again, the test to be met is what the reasonable owner would want to know, not what the reasonable veterinarian would disclose.

RESTRICTIONS IMPOSED BY THE PROFESSION

In addition to the broad provisions and regulations contained in the FDA and the NCA, the Veterinarians Act (VA) of Ontario (and similar legislation in other provinces) addresses the question of the extra-label use of drugs.

The regulations under the VA speak both to the standard of practice to be maintained by the practitioner and to the use and maintenance of drugs. The regulations are specific and must be adhered to; failure to abide by them can result in disciplinary proceedings.

Part III of the regulations deals with the use, dispensing, and storage of drugs; the extra-label use of drugs is not specifically addressed. However, the information contained on the manufacturer's label is deemed to be within your knowledge; consequently, you are deemed to know when an extra-label use occurs

Of more importance are the regulations contained in part II of the VA, which relate to practice standards and what actions may be regarded as professional misconduct in the context of extra-label drug use.

STANDARD OF PRACTICE

The extra-label use of a drug, in the absence of careful consideration and consultation on the part of the practitioner, could constitute professional misconduct. To fall within an acceptable practice standard, the use of a drug in a manner or in a dosage not contemplated by its manufacturer must be widely adopted by the profession. The veterinarian is obliged to consider how widespread the extra-label use of a drug is before prescribing and dispensing such a drug in such a fashion to a patient.

MISREPRESENTATIONS TO CLIENTS

Implicit in the off-label administration of a drug is the belief on the veterinarian's part that the use will be beneficial to the animal. Be careful that your belief does not lead you to tell a client that such a use will guarantee a particular result. On the contrary: you must tell the client that the use is extra-label, and disclose and explain the risks of such use. In addition, you must ensure that any claim you make is supportable by professional opinion.

Extra-label use, like other professional practices, is governed by the standard of "reasonableness." The CVO is mandated by the VA to issue a finding of unprofessional conduct if the practitioner fails to adhere to that standard of care.

DUTY TO THE PUBLIC

Extra-label drug use in an agricultural setting can result in drug residues that enter the food chain. Veterinarians have received increasing numbers of requests from farmers and others to prescribe medications or administer vaccinations without examining the animal. Very often such a request is made in the hope of saving money.

Whenever a veterinarian prescribes an extra-label usage of a drug, he or she must provide the client food producer with information concerning the animal's withdrawal from the drug and the consequences of the increased dosage or duration. Similarly, the veterinarian must provide information on the storage of drugs and on recordkeeping. These precautions are necessary if you are to meet the standard of care owed by the practitioner to the public generally.

In 1986, in *Buchan v. Ortho Pharmaceuticals (Canada) Ltd.* ((1986), 54 OR (2d) 92), the Ontario Court of Appeal effectively extended the doctrine of informed consent to the drug manufacturer. In that case it was held that the manufacturer had not fulfilled its duty of care when it failed to advise a doctor of the possibility of stroke in a patient who took oral contraceptives. The court held that the patient, as well, had to be advised. This case suggests that a veterinarian may be under a similar positive obligation to advise a food-producer client not only of the risks attached to the normal use of a drug, but of the risks associated with extra-label use, particularly withdrawal times and the possibility of residue.

Further, in some instances there may be sufficient evidence of causation to catch the veterinarian in the net of liability. A harmful residue that was not disclosed to a farmer and that is subsequently ingested by an end consumer can lead to the veterinarian's liability on the principle outlined in the *Ortho* decision. In summary, you must be very cautious in prescribing an extra-label use in food-producing animals, because potential litigants in a negligence action include the consuming public. As stated above, it is prudent to keep detailed records of your discussions with your clients, and to ensure that the off-label use is generally recognized by the profession to meet the standard of use by the reasonable practitioner.

From a practice-management perspective, it is wise to develop a good relationship with clients so as to avoid treating an animal without offering full disclosure. Do not give in to a client's insistence on the extra-label use of a drug because you fear the loss of that client's business. Despite the monetary value of drug sales, consenting to such demands will not be worth the legal problems that might subsequently arise.

CLIENT COMPLAINTS AND DISCIPLINE

Sometimes, despite your best efforts in practice and despite the effective management tools you have developed for your clinic, a medical procedure may not lead to a successful result. At a minimum, there is a likelihood that the client's expectations, reasonable or not, will not have been met, leaving the client disgruntled or otherwise unsatisfied. While these disputes can usually be resolved by you and your client through open discussion, sometimes the pet owner or farmer may feel that further action is necessary. Alternatively, you may be retained to act on behalf of an owner who has previously dealt with one of your colleagues, and it may become apparent to you that your colleague's actions are deserving of review by your province's regulatory body.

This aspect of veterinary practice management is regulated by provincial rules; owing to space limitations, a detailed review of each jurisdiction's regulations is impossible here. The discussion that follows is largely based on the laws and regulations in force in Ontario. Where it is appropriate, similar provisions in the legislation of other provinces are addressed.

PRACTICE POINT

As a member of your professional association, you are required by law to cooperate with any investigation undertaken by the profession's governing body. An uncooperative or unresponsive attitude may add to the severity of any sanctions imposed.

COMPLAINTS

Section 23 of the Veterinarians Act (VA) of Ontario provides for the establishment of a complaints committee of the College of Veterinarians of Ontario (CVO). Provisions in section 14 of the Nova Scotia Veterinary Medical Act and in section 19 of the Veterinarians Act of Saskatchewan, for example, establish similar committees to receive and act upon complaints from the public or the profession. In Ontario, the committee is normally made up of a panel of no fewer than three and not more than ten persons, of whom at least one is a member of the council of the regulatory body; the others are members of the association. To avoid the appearance of bias, any member of the complaints committee who is involved in the investigation of a member's conduct is generally prohibited from sitting as a member of the discipline committee that might later hear the case.

In Newfoundland and Labrador, it appears that jurisdiction in disciplinary matters is shared by the Newfoundland and Labrador Veterinary Licensing Board and the Newfoundland and Labrador Veterinary Medical Association. The council of the association consists of six persons, each of whom must be a member in good standing of the association. The council has the authority to make bylaws for the government and discipline of association members. The three-member disciplinary committee of the association may reprimand, censure, suspend, or expel any association member upon a finding of unprofessional conduct, negligence, or misconduct or upon a conviction of a criminal offence as designated in the bylaws. The committee will investigate the matter, conduct a hearing if necessary, and make a recommendation to council. The council must then make a final decision and notify the member of the decision. Within sixty days of receiving notice of the decision, the member may appeal the decision to a judge of the trial division of the Supreme Court of Newfoundland and Labrador.

While the licensing board also has the authority to deal with disciplinary matters, the regulations under the Veterinary Medical Act of Newfoundland and Labrador provide that any written complaint made to the board concerning a member of the association may be referred to the association's disciplinary committee. The board will await the disposition of the complaint by the association before exercising its own powers under the legislation. Thus it appears that the association has a form of paramountcy over the board when it comes to dealing with complaints.

Similarly, in Prince Edward Island a dual disciplinary authority is in place. The council of the Prince Edward Island Veterinary Medical Association has jurisdiction to discipline its members, and the licensing board has jurisdiction to deal with the discipline of licensees. The hearing process is similar to Ontario's; within thirty days of the hearing, the council must render a decision and notify the complainant and any other person the council deems advisable. Any appeal of the decision is to a judge of the Supreme Court of Prince Edward Island.

The Veterinarians Act of New Brunswick also provides for complaints and discipline committees to be established. Part VI of the act states that the council of the New Brunswick Veterinary Medical Association, upon receiving a complaint concerning a member, must cause an investigation to be carried out by the complaints committee if the complaint involves any allegation of professional misconduct, conduct unbecoming a member of the profession, incompetence, dishonesty, any suggestion of unfitness to practise, any breach of the act or bylaws, or any habit that renders the member unfit, incapable, or unsafe to practise veterinary medicine. An investigation can be launched if there are allegations that the member may be suffering from any "ailment or condition" that renders him or her incompetent to practise.

It is interesting to note that section 34(3) of the New Brunswick act provides that no complaint which, in substance, concerns fees or charges can be referred to the complaints committee. It appears that in that province the profession has determined that the better course of action is to permit the complainant to commence a court action for any compensation relating to fees. Another interesting aspect of the process in New Brunswick relates to the evidence to be adduced to the complaints committee. Under section 35(6) of the New Brunswick act, the committee can consider written evidence provided by the complainant or the member complained of. Part VII of the New Brunswick act deals with appeals from the decisions of the discipline committee. The first appeal is not to a court, but to the council of the Veterinary Medical Association, with a further right of appeal to the courts.

Any person is permitted to lodge a complaint against a member of the Veterinary Medical Association of Manitoba to the Veterinary Medical Board of Manitoba. The board is mandated to commence an investigation into the matter complained of. If it is satisfied that the complaint is frivolous, the board is required to dismiss the complaint and advise the complainant. In the event that the complaint is valid, the board then conducts an inquiry where appropriate evidence is reviewed.

In Ontario, the mandate of the complaints committee as set out in section 24 of the VA is to "consider and investigate complaints made by members of the public or members of the College regarding the conduct of a member or former member of the College." A written complaint must be filed with the registrar of the CVO, and the member or former member against whom the complaint is made must be notified of the complaint and given at least two weeks to submit an explanation in writing. In addition, the complaints committee is charged with a duty to examine or make all reasonable efforts to examine all documents relating to the complaint.

Upon reviewing a complaint, the committee may take one of three courses of action. First, it may direct that the matter be referred to the discipline committee in whole or in part, or it may refer the matter to the registrar in circumstances where the member's ability to continue practising may be impaired. Second, it can direct that the matter not be referred to the discipline committee or to the attention of the registrar. Third, it may exercise a broad power to "take such action as it considers appropriate in the circumstances that is not inconsistent with the [legislation]." In any event, any direction must be delivered in writing to the registrar. In the event that the matter is not being referred to either the registrar or the discipline committee, the complaints committee must state the reasons for taking that course of action.

In some circumstances the member against whom a complaint is made may be required to appear before the committee, and the committee may provide the member with advice concerning the member's practice of veterinary medicine.

Notice of any decision of the complaints committee must be given to the member by regular mail, together with notice that the member has the right to have the decision of the committee reviewed.

If the complainant or the member against whom the complaint is made is dissatisfied with the decision of the complaints committee (except a decision to refer the matter to the discipline committee), either party may advise the registrar of the CVO that he or she requests the Health Disciplines Board of Ontario to review the decision. All documents relating to the matter are then forwarded to the board and the decision of the complaints committee is reviewed. The board has the power to permit the complainant or the member to respond to the decision or otherwise state his or her case. These proceedings are generally held in private; however, upon the request of the member, the hearing may be held publicly, provided that the subject matter does not involve public security or the disclosure of intimate financial or personal matters.

As in other disciplinary proceedings, no person is permitted to make any audio or visual recording of the proceedings, and the member's name cannot be published unless the member consents to such publication or until the board has made its decision and is required to respond to the registrar.

In the event that the complaints committee has not dealt with a particular matter within 120 days after the complaint was made, the board has the power to require the committee to make the proper investigations. Then the committee must complete the ordered investigation within the next 120 days, failing which the board may commence its own investigations.

Like the complaints committee, the board has a legislated set of options to choose from in reaching its decisions: first, it may confirm the decision of the complaints committee; second, it may make recommendations to the complaints committee; third, it may require the complaints committee to take any action or proceeding available under the legislation. All decisions of the board must be in writing.

In the Northwest Territories, disciplinary matters are delegated to a board of inquiry consisting of two or more members appointed by the commissioner of the territorial government. The board is responsible for investigating any complaint made against a veterinary surgeon with respect to any violation of the applicable statute, or for "infamous, disgraceful or improper conduct." After completing its investigation, the board must report to the commissioner. If the board finds the practitioner to have committed the offence complained of, the commissioner may suspend or cancel the practitioner's licence.

DISCIPLINE

In Ontario, the discipline committee is made up of ten members of the council of the CVO, at least two of whom are appointed by the provincial cabinet. Three members of the committee constitute a quorum so long as one of them is the cabinet appointee. The decisions of the committee require a majority.

The findings of the discipline committee must be based solely on admissible evidence that is adduced at a hearing and on certain special matters that, by the rules of law, are admissible by notice. The member has the opportunity to examine before a hearing any written or documentary evidence that will be produced or given in evidence at the hearing. Special rules permit any party to call expert witnesses. The name of the expert, his or her address and qualifications, and the substance of his or her testimony must be provided to the other party at least ten days before the hearing. This requirement may be waived by the committee or allowed, provided that the other party consents.

PRACTICE POINT

Disciplinary proceedings are governed by the laws of fundamental justice, which are rooted in ensuring the fairness of the hearing. Strict rules of evidence, such as those that are in force in a court trial, may be relaxed somewhat in order to ensure that the parties' positions are fairly represented to the tribunal.

No member of the discipline committee may take part in any investigation leading up to the hearing, except in special circumstances. The discipline committee itself may seek independent legal advice apart from the advice granted to either of the parties to the hearing. Counsel for the committee is generally retained to advise on matters of the law of evidence and technical procedure. In the event that such advice is rendered, the nature of the advice given to the committee must be disclosed to the parties.

As in court proceedings, a transcript of the evidence given at a disciplinary hearing is made available to the parties. In this case, the parties to the hearing are the college itself and the member whose conduct is under scrutiny. The complainant is not a party to the hearing; rather, it is usual to have the complainant appear as a witness at the hearing.

As in hearings before the Health Disciplines Board, no audio or visual recording of the proceedings is permitted and no identification of the member may be published except with the consent of the party or after the discipline committee has rendered its decision.

In Alberta, under section 39 of the Veterinary Profession Act, all proceedings before the discipline committee are held in camera — that is, they are not open to the public. The strict rules of evidence that would apply in a court of law are relaxed for the purposes of the committee's proceedings.

The subject matter of a disciplinary hearing generally relates to allegations of professional misconduct or serious neglect on the part of a practitioner. These matters go to the committee not from the complaints committee but from the council or executive committee of the cvo or its equivalent.

PROFESSIONAL MISCONDUCT

A member of the CVO must be found guilty of professional misconduct by the discipline committee in four instances:

1. if the member has been found guilty of an offence relevant to the member's ability to practise veterinary medicine;

2. if the member's right or privilege to practise veterinary medicine under a federal or provincial law other than the VA has been restricted or withdrawn;

3. if there has been a finding of professional misconduct or serious neglect against the member by a veterinary authority in a jurisdiction other than Ontario; or

4. if the member has been found guilty of professional misconduct as defined in the regulations to the VA.

In Alberta, professional misconduct is defined as any act that is detrimental to the best interests of the public, contravenes the statutory code of ethics, harms the standing of the profession generally, displays a lack of knowledge in the practice of the profession, or displays a lack of knowledge in carrying out an undertaking of the profession. In Newfoundland a practitioner is guilty of professional misconduct if he or she is involved in any act or omission which, in the opinion of the discipline committee, amounts to an unjustifiable breach of duty to the public, a client, a patient, or any other member of the profession. The Newfoundland definition is extremely broad and open to subjective interpretations of the committee.

In Saskatchewan, section 24 of the Veterinarians Act broadly defines unprofessional conduct in the following terms: "Unprofessional conduct is a question of fact but any matter, conduct or thing, whether or not disgraceful or dishonourable, that is inimical to the best interests of the public or the members of the [Saskatchewan] association or tends to harm the standing of the profession of veterinary medicine is unprofessional conduct within the meaning of this Act." A definition of such latitude confers on the discipline committee a good deal of discretion in dealing with any conduct that is not in "the best interests of the public" or the profession.

The first appeal from a decision of the discipline committee is to the council of the Saskatchewan Veterinary Medical Association, with a subsequent appeal to the superior court of Saskatchewan, the Court of Queen's Bench.

In Ontario, the regulations provide that a veterinarian is guilty of professional misconduct in a number of statutorily defined circumstances. In the other common law provinces, similar types of provisions are found in the bylaws of the veterinary association as set out in the legislation. A discussion of the Ontario provisions encompasses a number of similar situations where disciplinary action may become an issue. A review of those circumstances indicates that professional misconduct can be categorized under eight separate headings.

Statutory Misconduct

Under section 17 of the regulations under the VA, a veterinarian can be found guilty of professional misconduct for a number of reasons that relate specifically to the terms of the VA itself. For instance, a veterinarian is guilty of misconduct if he or she participates in any activity that is inconsistent with the act or its regulations. In addition, as discussed in chapter 4, the mandate of the CVO is to grant specific types of licences; charges of professional misconduct can arise if one fails to abide by a condition of the licence or certificate of accreditation. The need to cooperate with the CVO in an investigation has already been highlighted; a practitioner may be guilty of professional misconduct if he or she fails to reply within a reasonable time to a written inquiry from the CVO. Charges of professional misconduct can also arise if one violates a broadly based regulation that dictates the need to act in a manner that cannot generally and reasonably be considered unprofessional conduct.

Practice Standards

As one might expect, the failure to maintain a high practice standard can result in a charge of professional misconduct. A general requirement to maintain the standard of practice of the profession is set out in the provincial regulations or bylaws. In addition, one must continue to provide professional services to an animal until the services are no longer required or until the client has had a reasonable opportunity to arrange for the services of another veterinarian. The veterinarian is prohibited from providing a service that is not reasonably necessary and reasonable. In addition, he or she must provide sufficient supervision of subordinates and cannot counsel any other person, other than a member of the CVO, to practise veterinary medicine. This last provision is important in large-animal practices, where the farmer client often administers medication or treatments under the direction of a veterinarian.

Client Communication

The failure to communicate effectively with a client is deemed to be professional misconduct. For example, a veterinarian must provide any report requested by a client within a reasonable time, and must maintain the confidentiality of communications. Professional misconduct can occur if a misrepresentation is made to a client or prospective client. If an animal has died unexpectedly or from an anaesthetic, you must advise the client of the availability of a necropsy through an independent veterinarian. Finally, it is clearly professional misconduct if you verbally or physically abuse a client.

A unique aspect of the Quebec Professional Code is that members of any profession, including veterinarians, are prohibited from refusing to provide services to a client because of "race, colour, sex, age, religion, national extraction or social origin of such person."

Fees

The veterinarian is prohibited from charging an excessive fee and from charging a fee for an unperformed service. It is misconduct to knowingly submit a false or misleading account to a client, to fail to issue a receipt upon request, to reduce or offer to reduce a fee for prompt payment, and to charge interest on an overdue account without notifying the client of that policy before providing service.

In Quebec, the Code of Ethics requires the practitioner to inform his or her client as soon as possible of the eventual cost of the operation and to seek the client's agreement in this regard. In addition, the practitioner is not permitted to withdraw services unless he or she has "sound and reasonable grounds" for so doing, including the loss of the client's confidence, the existence of a conflict of interest, or in response to a client's request to perform an illegal act. The Code of Ethics also requires the Quebec practitioner to "request and accept fair and reasonable fees." The veterinarian in Quebec must refrain from demanding payment in advance for services, but may request a preliminary payment for expenses that are likely to be incurred. The Code of Ethics dictates that "the veterinary surgeon must have exhausted all the other means at his [or her] disposal to obtain payment for fees." Sometimes it may be difficult for the practitioner to determine when "all the other means" have been exhausted.

Disposal

Veterinarians are under an obligation to dispose of an animal in accordance with the wishes of the client, provided that those wishes are in accordance with law and accepted veterinary standards of practice.

Conflict of Interest

Charges of professional misconduct may be filed against a practitioner who is in a conflict of interest. This topic is discussed in more detail in chapter 13.

Records

The failure to maintain accurate and up-to-date records may result in a finding of professional misconduct. In addition, faulty recordkeeping may seriously prejudice your defence in any civil claim against you for negligence. Falsifying a record also constitutes misconduct, as does signing or issuing a veterinary certificate or record without first ascertaining its accuracy.

Professional Courtesy

The regulations require that you treat your colleagues with respect and courtesy. You are prohibited from making a statement, orally or in writing, calculated to belittle or injure the professional reputation of a colleague. You must not treat an animal that is receiving veterinary services from another practitioner without notifying that practitioner. Similarly, you must advise the client that such uncoordinated treatment may place the animal at risk.

In addition to the foregoing, the regulations set out a test for determining when any of the actions described above, together with others, falls below an acceptable standard. Section 18 of the Ontario regulations dictates that a veterinarian must "exercise generally accepted standards of practice and procedures in the performance of veterinary services."

SERIOUS NEGLECT

A member is guilty of serious neglect if, in the opinion of the discipline committee, the member has displayed "in his or her professional care of an animal a lack of knowledge, skill or judgement or disregard for the welfare of the animal of a nature that demonstrates that [he or she] is unfit to engage in the practice of veterinary medicine," or, if fit, only under certain conditions imposed by the discipline committee. In other words, the committee may find that the veterinarian is fit to practise but only subject to certain restrictions imposed on his or her licence; for instance, the discipline committee may demand that the practitioner undertake and successfully complete a course of retraining or professional enhancement to upgrade his or her skills prior to performing certain types of surgery.

An interesting aspect of the Manitoba Veterinary Medical Act is that where incompetence is alleged, the board must find that the veterinarian's act or omission constitutes "gross negligence." Presumably, the threshold for a finding of gross negligence is higher than that for simple negligence. One might speculate on whether or not a finding of "incompetence" in Manitoba is the same as a finding of "serious neglect" in Ontario. The test in Ontario does not seem to require a finding of gross negligence to lead to a finding of "serious neglect."

PENALTIES

In the event that a veterinarian is found guilty by the provincial discipline committee of professional misconduct or serious neglect, the committee has the power to impose one or any combination of the following penalties:

1. revoke the licence to practise;

2. withdraw any specialist status;

3. suspend the licence to practise for a stated period;

4. impose conditions and limitations upon the licence;

5. impose a monetary fine;

6. reprimand the member; or

7. direct that the imposition of any penalty be suspended or postponed upon terms directed by the committee.

The circumstances in which a veterinarian's licence to practice would be revoked as a result of disciplinary action must be particularly grave. A 1968 Alberta case, *Re Roenisch and Alberta Veterinary Medical Association* (66 DLR (2d) 358), stands for the proposition that the acts of the practitioner must go beyond mere professional negligence; some degree of intent or turpitude must be evident in order to revoke the professional's licence to practise. In this case, the veterinarian apparently misdiagnosed a cat with a flu virus and allegedly bandaged a dog's foot so tightly that circulation was prevented and the dog was later destroyed. The Alberta Veterinary Medical Association reviewed the matter and ordered that the practitioner's name be struck from the register on the grounds of malpractice and unprofessional conduct. The veterinarian's appeal to the court was allowed and his name restored to the register on the basis that his actions, while perhaps negligent, lacked any intention to perform poorly.

The publication of the committee's findings can be a severe penalty for the practitioner. In the event that a fine is levied or a reprimand issued, the publication of the name of the member is often required in addition. In certain circumstances, the committee has the ability to direct the registrar not to publish the practitioner's name. Under the Quebec Professional Code, the regulatory body must publish an annual compilation of certain disciplinary decisions, omitting, where appropriate, the names of the members disciplined if an order banning publication has been made. Such a publication ban may be required if particularly sensitive evidence regarding the financial or emotional status of the practitioner has been adduced at the disciplinary hearing.

APPEALS FROM DECISIONS OF THE DISCIPLINE COMMITTEE

The decision of the committee and the penalty imposed are effective immediately, even if an appeal is launched, unless the court to which the appeal is directed orders otherwise, if the penalty includes revocation or suspension with or without conditions of the member's licence to practise upon a finding of serious neglect. A finding of professional misconduct and the subsequent penalty imposed do not take effect until the time to file an appeal has expired.

In Alberta, the first right of appeal is to the council of the Alberta Veterinary Medical Association, with a further appeal to the Court of Appeal of Alberta.

In Quebec, an appeal from a decision of the discipline committee is to a special board, the Professions Tribunal.

In Manitoba, the appeal is to the Court of Queen's Bench. The judge who hears the appeal may order that the costs of the appeal proceeding be paid by the unsuccessful party.

COSTS OF PROCEEDINGS

In some provinces, the penalties imposed by the disciplinary body include orders that an unsuccessful practitioner pay the costs of the investigations and/or proceedings of the regulatory body. In Ontario, the CVO is reviewing its approach, which currently does not permit the organization to make an award for costs.

The New Brunswick Veterinarians Act specifically provides that any of the complaints or discipline committees, the council of the New Brunswick Veterinary Medical Association, or the courts may order that the costs associated with their proceedings be paid by the member against whom the complaint was made or by the complainant. Costs are not to be ordered from the member in cases where the complaint is completely dismissed without any adverse orders against the member, or by the complainant if the complaint was, in the opinion of the tribunal, warranted.

Similarly, the bylaws of the Nova Scotia Veterinary Medical Association provide that the council may, if a complaint is proved, order that the member reimburse the association for all or a part of the costs of the disciplinary proceeding and the preceding investigation, together with reasonable fees and disbursements of any legal counsel engaged by the association.

Like some of the Maritime provinces, Saskatchewan also provides for the payment of costs by the unsuccessful party in a disciplinary hearing. Under the Saskatchewan Veterinarians Act, the costs include "the expenses of the professional conduct committee and discipline committee."

The Alberta legislation also provides for the payment of costs by the unsuccessful party. Section 13(1) of the general regulations to the Alberta legislation contains a catalogue of costs that may be recovered, including "any transportation, accommodation and living expenses paid to a person conducting a preliminary investigation," along with an honorarium. The costs associated with obtaining a transcript of the evidence and witness fees are also recoverable. Room rentals, legal fees charged by counsel for the association, and the costs associated the service of any documents can amount to an expensive bill for the unsuccessful party.

Similarly, the Manitoba Veterinary Medical Act provides that any unsuccessful practitioner in a disciplinary hearing before the province's Board of Inquiry may be subject to an order to pay all or any of the costs and expenses incurred by the board relating to the investigation and subsequent hearing.

British Columbia is one of the few jurisdictions that have dealt with the second issue relating to the costs of disciplinary action: that is, if a complaint is found to be without merit, does the member complained of receive compensation to offset the costs he or she has incurred in defending the claim? Section 16 of the Veterinarians Act of British Columbia gives the Council of the British Columbia Veterinary Medical Association the discretion to make an order to pay out of funds generally at its disposal the costs incurred by any person against whom a complaint has been made that is found to have been "frivolous and vexatious." Such claims probably will be limited to cases where the complaint was wholly without merit from the outset, and not to those cases where a complaint has been dismissed by the discipline committee. A similar provision is found in Ontario.

Could the professional association's ability to order an unsuccessful party to pay the costs of the proceedings give rise to an appearance of bias or partiality? This issue was dealt with by the New Brunswick Court of Queen's Bench in *McAllister v. New Brunswick Veterinary Medical Association* (71 NBR (2d) 109) in 1986. In that case, a veterinarian had been found guilty of professional misconduct and had applied to the court before a penalty was imposed to enjoin the proceedings on the ground of bias. That argument was rejected by the court, which found that although the council had the power to award costs against the practitioner, it did not raise an apprehension of bias necessary to halt the proceedings. While other provincial courts are not required to follow this line of reasoning, it seems that this is the law in Canada on this issue at present.

In Quebec, section 151 of the Professional Code states that the discipline committee has the "power to condemn the complainant or the respondent to pay the costs, including the cost of recording."

IMPAIRMENT

Under section 33 of the VA in Ontario, a board of inquiry may be appointed by the executive committee of the CVO in the event that the registrar "receives information leading the registrar to believe that a member of the College may be impaired." In effect, the registrar conducts an investigation "as he or she considers appropriate" and makes a report to the executive committee, which may, after giving notice to the member, appoint the board of inquiry. This three-member panel is made up of at least two members of the CVO and a cabinet appointee.

The board of inquiry then conducts its own investigation, which may include directing the member to undergo physical or mental examination. In the event that the member refuses to undergo such an examination, the board has a sweeping power to order that the member's licence be suspended until he or she complies.

The board of inquiry must then report to the executive committee of the CVO and provide a copy of its report to the member. The executive committee may then refer the matter to the registration committee of the CVO to hold a hearing, and may suspend the member's licence until the final decision of the registration committee is made. In these cases the central issue is whether or not the ability of the member to practise veterinary medicine is impaired. Medical evidence is usually the hallmark of such a hearing.

PRACTICE POINT

A finding of impairment for a partner in a veterinary practice can lead to a revocation of his or her licence to practise; therefore, any partnership agreement should include a provision that the agreement can be terminated upon any suspension or revocation of the licence to practise of a partner. Since that partner will no longer contribute professionally to the practice, you must determine whether or not his or her financial interest in the practice should continue.

The registration committee must then report and determine whether or not the member's ability is impaired. If impairment is found, the committee may revoke the member's licence, suspend the licence indefinitely or for a certain period of time, or attach conditions to the licence as it considers appropriate. These proceedings normally take place in private.

Section 36 of the Veterinarians Act of New Brunswick also authorizes the discipline committee of the New Brunswick Veterinary Medical Association to require a member to submit to "physical or mental health examinations by such qualified person or persons as the Committee may designate." In the event that the member fails to submit to the examination or that its finding is unsatisfactory to the committee, the committee may, without further notice, suspend the member's registration and licence. The New Brunswick act specifies that such an examination is to "determine whether the member has adequate skill and knowledge to practise veterinary medicine."

Similar provisions are contained in the Professional Code of Quebec and relate not only to veterinarians but to most professions in that province. Section 48 dictates that the Bureau of a professional organization may order a medical examination of a person who is a member where it has reason to believe his or her physical or mental condition is incompatible with the practice of the profession. Such an examination is conducted by a panel of three physicians: one appointed by the Bureau, one by the person to be examined, and the third by the other two. In the event that the member refuses to submit to an examination or that the report is negative,then the bureau may strike the member from the roll, restrict the member's practice, or suspend the member from practice. A decision may be appealed to the Quebec Professions Tribunal.

COURT APPEALS

Any decision of the disciplinary committee, the registration committee, or other committees of the provincial regulatory bodies may be appealed to an appropriate court of law. The court may affirm or rescind the earlier decision, and may exercise all of the powers that the relevant committee itself could have exercised. In other words, the court can substitute its own decision for the decision of the committee appealed from.

INVESTIGATION

The registrar of the provincial regulatory body may investigate the conduct of a member if, in the opinion of the registrar, there are reasonable grounds for believing that a member has committed an act of professional misconduct or serious neglect, or that there is cause to refuse to issue or renew, or to suspend, a licence. Such an investigation usually can be made only with the approval of the executive committee. An investigator is appointed and a report on the investigation is made to the registrar.

The investigator may examine the member's practice. Upon presentation of the appointment issued by the registrar, the investigator may enter the practice at any reasonable time and make reasonable inquiries of any person. The investigator may also view any documents relevant to the investigation. If necessary, a warrant may be sworn out before a justice of the peace in furtherance of the investigation to permit entry to premises. Every member of a provincial veterinary association is required to co-operate with such an investigation.

The investigator's report is to be made available to the executive of the provincial body or to such other committee as the registrar deems appropriate. Presumably, further inquiries and hearings may follow such an investigation.

FINANCIAL ASSISTANCE IN PROSECUTING MEMBERS

In Nova Scotia bylaws, any veterinary member of the provincial association can seek the assistance of the association in prosecuting any practitioner for actions contrary to the Nova Scotia Veterinary Medical Act. The complaining member can present a written statement to the registrar concerning the nature of the evidence that can be obtained to secure a conviction. The registrar can then take the matter up with the council of the association to determine what assistance, if any, can be granted. In this manner, members of the association can ask for help in prosecuting anyone, member or non-member, who practises veterinary medicine contrary to the Nova Scotia laws.

The bylaws of the Saskatchewan Veterinary Medical Association provide that any legal action commenced against a member may be defended with the assistance of the association. A practitioner may make a written statement to the secretary of the association, who must immediately inform the other members of the council. The council then decides what, if any, assistance can be given to the member who is defending the action. A member must post a $100 good faith deposit towards the expenses of the association, which can be returned if not required.

PERSONAL PLANNING

12

So far, much of our discussion has related to the use of effective manage-ment tools so as to maximize the creation of wealth. In this chapter we will look at the law relating to the distribution of that wealth between spouses upon separation or divorce, and among beneficiaries upon the death of the practitioner. These matters fall almost exclusively within provincial juris-diction. The discussion that follows is based on Ontario law; the reader is advised to consult directly with his or her professional advisers to ascertain the provisions in force in other provinces.

FAMILY LAW

In Ontario, family law has undergone substantial reform in the last twenty years. Previously, the usual result of a marriage breakdown was that one spouse (normally the husband) retained income-earning ability, together with much of the marital property. The law recognized the plight of the de-pendent spouse (normally the wife) through such legislation as the Deserted Wives and Children's Maintenance Act and the Dower Act. To-day, however, men and women are equal before the law, and upon marriage breakdown or death their positions are equalized insofar as their as prop-erty is concerned. The first major piece of legislation to address the problem was the 1978 Family Law Reform Act, which divided family as-sets. In 1986 the act was revamped to include non-family assets, such as a spouse's business or partnership.

SCOPE OF LEGISLATION

The Ontario Family Law Act (FLA) governs such matters as the support of spouses and children, the division of property, and the creation of domestic contracts, including marriage contracts, separation agreements, and cohabitation agreements.

PRACTICE POINT

The effect of separation or divorce on an individual practitioner or on the partners of the practice can be substantial, given the relative value of the assets that make up the practice. Some cases have suggested that a spouse who assisted a professional in obtaining a degree may be entitled to an interest in the value of the practice upon dissolution of marriage.

The FLA is principally designed to deal with marriage breakdown, but also addresses the disposition of property following the death of a spouse. Bear in mind that there are many exceptions and twists to this complex statute, and that generalizations are difficult to apply to a specific situation. Many people have heard stories, for example, about a common law spouse who brings about the downfall of a practice or business. These anecdotal reports usually have little basis in fact. The FLA addresses two separate issues, which often become confused: one is the division of property; the other is a spouse's entitlement to support, whether a continuing periodic payment owing to a dependency, or a lump sum payment.

The FLA acknowledges that marriage is an economic as well as a social and emotional partnership. The preamble to the act reads as follows:

> Whereas it is desirable to encourage and strengthen the role of the family; and whereas for that purpose it is necessary to recognize the equal position of spouses as a form of a partnership; and whereas in support of such recognition it is necessary to provide in law for the orderly and equitable settlement of the affairs of the spouses upon the breakdown of the partnership, and to provide for other mutual obligations in family relationships, including equitable sharing by parents of responsibility for their children ...

Note the reference to the breakdown of the "partnership" as opposed to the breakdown of the marriage. The scope of the so-called partnership is all-embracing in its concepts of the sharing of assets for the benefit of the marriage and the distribution of those assets upon breakdown. As mentioned above, there is no distinction between family and non-family assets.

For property division purposes, people who are legally married, whether before or after 1986, are affected by the new property division rules. Unmarried persons are not affected by the rules relating to property division, as discussed below.

DIVISION OF ASSETS

The FLA does not provide for the actual physical division of property; rather, it provides for the division of the "value" of the property. Should one spouse have assets of greater value than the other spouse's assets, the assets are equalized. Although the court has the power to order that a specific asset be transferred in satisfaction of an equalization payment, in most cases the equalization is accomplished by the payment of funds equal to the share of the value determined.

EXEMPT PROPERTY

Certain types of property are exempt from the equalization provisions. The first of these is property (for example, a veterinary clinic) owned by a spouse before the date of marriage. It is often difficult to determine the value of such property; it may be necessary to consult a professional veterinary valuator.

The second exemption is a gift or inheritance received from a third party during the marriage. This is perhaps the most difficult value to calculate, in that gifts often take the form of money, which is assimilated into family income and is thereafter unidentifiable. For the purposes of the exemption, the asset or the money must exist at the time of death or separation. If the money can be traced to a specific asset, the value of that asset at the time of the gift can operate as a proper exemption. Note that it is the value at the time of the gift, not at the time of separation or death that is relevant.

A third exemption is the income earned from, or a capital gain in, a gift or inheritance, provided that the donor specifically stated that the income or gain was not to be shared with the recipient's spouse. This important exemption should be borne in mind when making a bequest in a will: one can never predict how a beneficiary's marriage will weather the years.

Yet another exemption is a court award for damages for personal injuries, or for loss of guidance, care, and companionship as a result of the death of a family member. This exemption was included in the legislation because such damages are highly personal to the individual and are not a proper subject matter for division.

An exemption is also allowed for proceeds from a life insurance policy paid to the spouse on the death of an insured person. This provision is similar to the gift exemption set out above.

The final exemption is property that the spouses have agreed, by way of a domestic contract, is not to be included in the division of property upon marriage breakdown or death. This exemption is discussed later in this chapter.

CALCULATION OF A DIVISION OF PROPERTY

The following table illustrates a typical division of property upon marriage breakdown.

	Spouse A	*Spouse B*
Value of property owned at time of marriage	$23,000	$7,000
Debts and liabilities at time of marriage	(4,000)	(1,000)
Net value of property at time of marriage	$19,000	$6,000
Property owned at time of separation	$50,000	$12,000
Debts and liabilities at time of separation	(8,000)	(2,000)
Net value of property at time of separation	$42,000	$10,000
Increase in value of property during marriage	$23,000	$4,000
Inheritance received	(10,000)	
Proceeds from parent's life insurance policy		(2,000)
Net value of family property	$13,000	$2,000

Spouse B's net value of family property is deducted from that of spouse A. The result is divided between the two parties: $13,000 – $2,000 x 50% = $5,500. Note that each party's debts are deducted from his or her property at the time of separation and at the time of marriage.

UNEQUAL DIVISION

In certain unusual situations one spouse can force an unequal division of property when an equal division would be unconscionable. The courts can order an unequal division in the following situations:

1. failure by a spouse to disclose debts and liabilities at the time of marriage;

2. if a spouse has been reckless or has in bad faith incurred debts that drastically reduce the net family property;

3. if a spouse intentionally or in a reckless fashion reduces the value of his or her property;

4. if the spouses have lived together for a period of less than five years; and

5. if there is a written agreement between the spouses that does not constitute a domestic contract.

MATRIMONIAL HOME

The family residence receives special treatment in the FLA, probably because it is normally a family's largest and most important asset. A veterinary practice, or any other business, does not have the same status. The family home is always brought into the calculation of net family property, regardless of the fact that it may have been inherited or purchased from damages awarded for a personal injury suffered by one of the spouses. This is a difficult area of the law. For example, consider a case in which spouse A had $100,000 at the time of marriage. The day after the marriage, he bought a home with spouse B, using the money. Later, when they separate, he will be entitled to a $100,000 deduction from his family assets. If the home had been purchased before the marriage, and spouse B had simply moved into the home, no deduction would be allowed, because the home has a special status pursuant to the act.

To complicate things further, the right to possession of the matrimonial home is deemed to be equal as between the spouses regardless of ownership, and cannot be dealt with in a marriage contract. It remains to be seen how one can remove the other spouse from the home after separation, although the FLA does provide for an application for exclusive possession. With respect to a division of property the conduct of either spouse is irrelevant, although it may have some relevance with respect to an award for periodic support.

EQUALIZATION AND THE VETERINARY PRACTICE

The FLA recognizes that if an immediate payment for equalization would seriously impair the operation of a veterinary practice, the court has discretion to award the non-owning spouse a share of the profits in the practice or to transfer an ownership interest to him or her. (It is not clear how this could be done when the veterinary legislation in most provinces require that all owners be veterinarians.) The court can also permit the spouse who must make the equalizing payment to defer it for as long as ten years.

VALUING THE PRACTICE

One of the most contentious issues in attempting to deal with financial statements for family law purposes is the valuation of the practice. Wide discrepancies in valuation can be justified by different appraisers, who must place a value on goodwill, inventories or drugs and accessories, and accounts receivable. Although the drafters of the FLA attempted to eliminate as much potential for litigation as possible, valuation disputes must sometimes be settled finally by a court. For this reason, it is important that the partners in a veterinary practice set out a clear valuation method for the practice in a written partnership agreement. Although it is not always binding, such a formula provides guidance for the judge. (A typical form of business valuation formula is set out in appendix R.) This topic is discussed in more detail below, under the heading "Domestic Contracts."

COMMON LAW SPOUSES

Common law spouses have no property rights under the FLA, regardless of the length of cohabitation. However, property division and support entitlement are two different issues, and a common law spouse, if dependent upon the other common law spouse, may bring an application for support under the FLA after three years of continuous cohabitation (or a lesser period if a child is born of the relationship). This form of relationship may also give rise to a property claim under the doctrine referred to as "resulting trusts." The rationale for such an action is that a person, while living with another, helped in the home or business to such an extent that the value was increased, and therefore the person should share in the value upon death or separation. These legal actions are becoming more common, and the courts are often sympathetic to such applications. An example of a court award in this area would be the case of the common law wife who stayed at home and reared the common law husband's children, painted his home, wallpapered, cooked, and otherwise supported the man. On the basis of the work performed during the relationship, the court held that the spouse was entitled to a payment for her labours.

DOMESTIC CONTRACTS

Scope of the Contract

The provisions of the FLA apply in the absence of a domestic contract. In the contract, the parties specify their respective rights and obligations during marriage, on separation, on divorce, or even on death. They may agree that the practice owned by one spouse is not to be included in that spouse's net family property. They may agree upon future support obligations (again with some exceptions, including support of children); in fact, they can agree upon any matters they wish to settle at the time of the execution of the agreement or upon the happening of a future event. Two exceptions are those mentioned above; the possession of the matrimonial home (not its ownership) and the right of custody of or access to their children. A sample domestic contract is reproduced in appendix s.

PRACTICE POINT

While the suggestion of the necessity of a domestic contract can be an emotional issue, the need for effective practice management dictates that you at least be aware of the risks of not having an agreement concerning the division of assets on matrimonial breakdown.

The Domestic Contract in Relation to the Practice

One of the objectives of your professional practice is to allow the clinic to carry on without interference from a spouse of a partner. You will also wish to maintain the confidentiality of the practice's financial affairs, which may be compromised by a partner's separation from his or her spouse. The separating partner's obligation to make a full financial disclosure includes the financial affairs of the practice. A separation may also involve an appraiser's poring over the financial statements of several years to review the receivables, inventory, etc. The appraiser will attempt to come up with a value for the practice. "Value" is not defined in the FLA. Market value is often used, but is that different from fair market value? If the criterion is fair market value, does that mean the value of the assets or the value of the business as a going concern? These are matters yet to be determined by the courts.

As mentioned above, it is usually a good idea to include in the partnership agreement a formula by which the value of the practice can be computed when necessary. However, you should be aware of some possible pitfalls. For example, a valuation determined pursuant to a provision in a partnership agreement might not be binding on a partner's spouse, since the spouse is not a party to the agreement and therefore cannot be said to have consented to the valuation provisions. While it is possible for a spouse to be made party to a partnership agreement, such a step could mean that the spouse would be deemed to have a proprietary interest in the practice. Alternatively, the spouse might later argue that he or she had so little knowledge of the business and the agreement that the signing constituted a nullity. To minimize the likelihood of such an event, the spouse must have independent legal advice before signing, and the lawyer who advises him or her should be fully aware of the nature of the practice and the terms of the agreement.

A better tactic is to require, in the partnership agreement, that all partners and their spouses enter into domestic contracts that exempt the partnership from the net family property. This arrangement is likely to satisfy the partners, but possibly not the spouses. In that event, legal advisers may wish to draft a kind of "compensating" provision in a domestic contract — for example, one that makes the matrimonial home the sole property of the non-veterinarian spouse, or one that permits an award of support based on the veterinarian's profits over a number of years.

The issue of equalization versus the protection of the veterinary practice is a complex one, and is best resolved in advance, early in the life of the practice. Although it is never easy to raise the topic of a domestic contract with one's spouse-to-be, the formation of such a contract can be most easily rationalized when a new practice is being formed.

DEATH OF A SPOUSE

The FLA provisions relating to marriage breakdown also apply to a spouse's death, where the deceased spouse did not provide one-half of the net family property to the surviving spouse. (In addition, the Succession Law Reform Act of Ontario contains provisions similar to the support provisions of the FLA.) For example, consider the situation where a parent, who has married for the second time, wishes to provide in his or her will for the children of the first marriage. Assume that a husband has three children from a former marriage, and leaves one-quarter of his estate to his new spouse and one-quarter to each of his children. The surviving new spouse may choose between abiding by the provisions set out in the deceased's will and receiving entitlement to an equalizing payment (based on the same calculations of net family property described earlier) under the FLA. (The valuation date for the calculation of the equalizing payment is the day before the spouse's death.)

The surviving spouse has six months to make the election between the will and the equalizing payment. Once again the solution is a domestic contract whereby the parties agree that upon death no elections will be made, and the surviving spouse will be satisfied with whatever provision is made in the deceased's will.

Given the complexities of the FLA, the possible intrusions of common law spouses, and the further imposition of the formula for distribution of an estate, it is important to ensure that your affairs are put in order in accordance with your circumstances.

ESTATE PLANNING

Each practitioner must ensure that the wealth created by the effective management of his or her veterinary practice is preserved for the purposes the practitioner desires. An important part of wealth preservation is the passing of the wealth to children and others upon the practitioner's death. An effective estate plan can ensure that all personal objectives of practice management are achieved.

INTESTATE SUCCESSION

When no will exists, either because the deceased has made no will or because a will is invalid, the estate is acquired by his or her heirs through intestate succession. In Ontario, the Succession Law Reform Act (SLRA) provides for the distribution of your estate if you die intestate. This means that the estate is distributed pursuant to the statute, without regard to your personal wishes:

1. If your spouse survives and no children are alive at the time of your death, your spouse receives the entire estate.

2. If your spouse survives together with one or more children, your spouse is entitled to a preferential share of the estate to a value of $75,000, with the remainder of the estate divided among your spouse and children in equal shares.

3. If your spouse does not survive you but your children do survive you, the estate is divided equally among your children.

4. If no spouse or children survive you, the estate is divided among family members in order of closeness of blood connection, including parents, siblings, nieces and nephews, and other next of kin.

5. If no family members survive you, your estate is distributed to the provincial government through a legal doctrine called escheats.

It is unlikely that these line of intestate succession will coincide with your specific plans for distribution.This is the primary reason why the development of a carefully considered estate plan is of vital importance in the preservation and distribution of your wealth.

PRACTICE POINT

The continuity of ownership of your practice can be addressed in your will. The practice may be the most significant asset in the estate; it is incumbent on the practitioner to develop an effective estate plan to make provision for beneficiaries. Do not procrastinate. The cost of a simple will is small in comparison with the grave consequences of not having a will.

TESTATE SUCCESSION

Testate succession is the acquisition of rights or property by a will. The concept of "testamentary freedom" dictates that you are free to distribute your estate in virtually any manner you choose.

DRAFTING A WILL

It is beyond question that one of the most important documents you will sign during your lifetime is your will. Your will dictates how your estate plan is to be carried out; accordingly, it is crucial that your will be clearly drafted so as to ensure the certainty you require in passing your wealth to your beneficiaries. A thoughtful and careful review of your estate plan is necessary if the will is to reflect your wishes accurately. The will must speak for you at a time when you are not present to give directions or render interpretations.

There are three main components in the preparation of a will: first, the appointment of executors, the persons who have been chosen by you to administer your estate; second, instructions to your executors as to the manner in which you want your estate disposed of; third, the granting of specific powers to your executors so that they may effectively administer your estate and carry out your wishes. Among other things, you may wish to appoint guardians for minor beneficiaries, provide instructions for your funeral arrangements, and establish forms of trusts for financial assets that may not be disposed of immediately.

Appointment of Executors

It is obvious that the person or persons whom you appoint as executors of your estate should be persons whom you trust implicitly to carry out your wishes as set out in your will. In addition, it is helpful if the executors have some knowledge of the location of your assets. Executors are often family members; however, you may appoint a trust firm or a trusted business or professional associate to fulfil this task.

A good planning technique is to appoint alternative executors of your estate in the event that your primary executor predeceases you or declines the appointment. In many cases, the primary executor is one's spouse; in that case the appointment of an alternative executor enables you to avoid redrafting your will if your spouse predeceases you.

Executors are charged in law with a fiduciary or trust relationship to act in the best interests of the estate and not on behalf of their own self-interest or in the interest of any particular beneficiary.

Disposition of Estate

Wills normally provide for three types of dispositions: legacies, bequests, and the distribution of the residue of the estate.

Legacies are specific gifts of money directed to be paid out of your estate to a person or institution of your choosing. The estate is charged with the obligation of converting assets into money for the payment of those legacies.

A bequest is similar to a legacy, except that it deals with the delivery to a beneficiary of a specific item of personal property. For instance, a family heirloom may be directed to be delivered to another family member. Similarly, items of aesthetic or personal appeal, such as jewellery, coin collections, stamp collections, and paintings, may be the subjects of bequests. A veterinarian may wish to pass on a library of professional texts to an associate in practice.

Those assets not previously disposed of through a bequest or legacy are deemed to fall into the balance of the estate, or the residue. A properly drafted will should contain a specific direction as to the disposition of the residue; the failure to include such a provision will result in the will's being partially invalid, as it fails to deal with all of the remaining assets of the estate. Often the residue is passed on to a spouse or other family members. In the event that those family members are under the ages of majority, it is advisable to establish a trust to maintain a fund until the beneficiary attains the age specified by you in your will.

Powers of Executors

You should give your executors the powers necessary to effectively administer your estate. Among other things, you should provide a power to invest funds of the estate for distribution, and the discretionary power to sell or retain assets. A clause such as the latter gives the executors the ability to take advantage of a favourable market in which to sell an asset in the future.

FORMAL VALIDITY OF WILLS

The signing of a will is subject to specific rules under the SLRA and the Wills Act in Ontario. The will must be signed by its maker (the testator or testatrix) and the signing must be witnessed by two persons who are present at the time the testator or testatrix signs it. If these rules are not followed, the will is invalid.

HOLOGRAPH WILLS

In Ontario, a will written in the handwriting of the testator (a holograph will) is a valid will, even if it is not witnessed. The will must be *entirely* in the testator's handwriting; it cannot be merely a "fill in the blank" document purchased from a stationery store.

CLAUSES CONCERNING ANIMALS

Veterinarians will be especially concerned to provide for the continued welfare of animals. Appendix T sets out various clauses dealing with the continued care and maintenance of pets and other animals.

REVOCATION

A will is automatically revoked and of no further validity upon the happening of any one of the following events:

1. marriage;

2. the making of a new will;

3. a written notice of revocation; or

4. the burning or tearing of it with the intention of destruction.

With respect to marriage, the SLRA states that a will made in contemplation of marriage and expressly described as such is not revoked upon the subsequent marriage.

ESTATE ADMINISTRATION

The scope of this text does not permit a detailed discussion of the administration procedures of an estate; however, a general overview of estate administration may be helpful.

Upon the death of the testator or testatrix, a review of the location and extent of the deceased's assets takes place. Executors should take special note of any assets that are owned jointly with other persons. Joint assets such as bank accounts or family residences do not become assets of the estate; by operation of law, the interest of the deceased owner automatically passes to the surviving owner. All other assets are to be identified and secured by the executors.

Next, the executors must determine whether court approval of the will and the administration of the estate is required through an application for letters probate from the appropriate provincial court. Depending on the value of the estate, the nature of the assets involved, and the number and location of beneficiaries, an application for probate is made so as to assure the validity of the will and to obtain court approval of the appointment of executors. In some cases, the completion of the estate administration is court-approved by having the executors pass the accounts of the estate before a judge, who reviews the administration duties of the executor.

ESTATE FREEZES

Because veterinarians in some jurisdictions are currently not permitted to incorporate the professional aspect of their practices, the value of a type of tax planning commonly referred to as an "estate freeze" is somewhat weakened; however, this vehicle for tax savings may be appropriate in the case of operating corporations that are permitted under provincial laws, and holding corporations that own the veterinary assets.

In its simplest form, an estate freeze is carried out when a taxpayer desires to "freeze" the value of his or her interest in the assets at a fixed time during his or her lifetime, with a view to having any increase in value accrue to beneficiaries (usually children) during their lifetimes. For the veterinarian, the most popular asset for which the "freeze" is appropriate is that of the real estate from which the practice is carried on; generally, that type of asset appreciates in value. In this context, real estate is a capital property for tax purposes which will give rise to a deemed disposition on the death of the owner. Prior to death, the owner can freeze the value of the real estate by converting the shares of the corporation that owns the real estate to a share that has a fixed value, while issuing new shares to beneficiaries. The increase in value of the real estate from the date of the freeze then accrues to the other beneficiaries until the shares held by them are sold or otherwise disposed of.

OTHER ESTATE-PLANNING TECHNIQUES

Several simple estate-planning techniques can be initiated during your lifetime.

Joint Ownership

The law of property dictates that assets, both personal property and real estate, may be owned jointly by a number of individuals. Upon the death of one joint owner ("joint tenant"), the interest of the deceased passes automatically, by operation of law, to the surviving joint tenant. Those assets that otherwise would pass by one's will may be distributed automatically through the right of survivorship.

PRACTICE POINT

The placing of assets in joint ownership can be an effective estate-planning tool; however, careful thought must go into such transfers. The imprudent transfer of assets can sometimes lead to a thwarting of a deceased's testamentary intention.

Plan Designations

Financial contracts such as insurance policies and RRSPs provide for the designation of a beneficiary of the financial benefit that accrues as a result of the contract. By designating a beneficiary, one simplifies the administration of an estate and avoids the accrual to the estate of unnecessary income for which tax would be payable.

Remember that the designation of a beneficiary through a financial contract is not necessarily final; the SLRA permits the owner to designate a person to benefit from many pension plans created after March 31, 1978.

Tax Havens

In the past, much was heard about the potential of moving assets to other jurisdictions so as to avoid the imposition of income taxes accruing from the assets. In most cases, such a plan cannot be implemented without triggering a "departure tax," which is imposed under the Income Tax Act when a Canadian resident changes his or her residency. In effect, capital properties are deemed to have been disposed of at their fair market value on the date of departure, thus giving rise to a capital gain or loss.

POWER OF ATTORNEY

Some mental and physical ailments can be so debilitating as to render you incompetent to act on your own behalf. One simple and inexpensive planning tool is the appointment of an attorney (meaning a person who is authorized to act for you) who can sign documents on your behalf and manage your financial affairs. Your solicitor can insert effective safeguards in the document to avoid abuse.

LIVING WILLS

While there is as yet no clear law on the subject in many provinces, many persons are requesting the preparation of living wills, which authorize medical authorities and family members to cease life support in cases where there is no reasonable expectation of a recovery. These documents are referred to as "health care directives" in some jurisdictions. The Ontario government has indicated its desire to provide legislative assistance in this highly emotional area. At the very least, those living wills presently in existence provide good evidence of the maker's intentions if a judicial application is made to cease life support.

PROFESSIONAL ETHICS

Most self-governing professions are guided by rules of ethics in their practices to ensure that the public is protected from the unscrupulous or incompetent practitioner. In many instances, a breach of the rules of ethics will lead to a similar breach of the laws and regulations governing the profession. The practitioner's ethical obligations are expressed in the Veterinarian's Oath, which is reproduced in appendix U.

STATUTORY CODES OF ETHICS

In some provinces, the legislation governing the practice of veterinary medicine includes codes of ethics either in the statute itself or in the accompanying regulations. The statutory codes may form the basis for misconduct proceedings when the ethical rules are breached.

Under section 87 of the Professional Code of Quebec, the Bureau must establish a code of ethics, by way of regulations, "governing the general and special duties of the professional towards the public, his clients and his profession, particularly the duty to discharge his professional obligations with integrity." The Corporation Professionelle des Médecins Vétérinaire du Québec has amended the code of ethics over the years. The code is divided into separate divisions dealing with veterinarians' duties to the public, their clients, the profession, and their patients. Many of these duties are similar to those established in the common law provinces. One unique aspect of the Quebec code of ethics is the requirement (in section 3.01.04) that the veterinary surgeon establish a relationship of mutual trust with his or her client. Presumably such a requirement is implicit in the codes of other jurisdictions.

In New Brunswick a code of ethics is set out in bylaw 14 of the New Brunswick Veterinary Medical Association. The "Rules of Professional

Conduct" are divided into three categories: responsibilities to the client; responsibilities to the profession; and responsibilities to society. Among other things, the veterinarian in New Brunswick is mandated by the bylaw to practise veterinary medicine to the best of his or her ability and to ensure that his or her conduct towards clients is above reproach. Confidentiality of records must be maintained, and practitioners are required to continue to educate themselves and to "adjust to modern concepts of veterinary medicine." The member shall "first of all be a good citizen" and shall commit no act that would reflect unfavourably on the profession. The practitioner is required to "build a professional reputation based on ability and integrity" and is not to belittle the professional standing of another member. A second veterinarian in a case shall make an effort to consult and co-operate with the former veterinarian to ensure the client's confidence in the profession. According to the New Brunswick rules, it is unethical to accept a fee from both the seller and the buyer relating to any pre-purchase inspection completed by the practitioner. Finally, the practitioner must not contravene any federal, provincial, or municipal law in the course of conducting his or her practice. The New Brunswick rules are quite broad and subjective. Each alleged breach must be reviewed on the basis of its own facts.

The bylaws of the Newfoundland and Labrador Veterinary Medical Association set out a code of ethics to be used as a "general guide to the behaviour expected of members of the Association by the Disciplinary Committee." While many of the provisions are the same as those found in other jurisdictions, some are unique. For example, the practitioner must have a general deportment "characterizing the personal behaviour of a lady or gentleman." He or she must "first of all be a good citizen" and be a leader in movements to promote community welfare. The term "unprofessional conduct" is defined as any act or omission which, in the opinion of the disciplinary committee, amounts to an unjustifiable breach of duty to the public, a client, a patient, or another member of the profession. "Negligence" is defined as any act or omission that falls below the standard of a reasonable degree of skill and care to be exercised by a veterinarian. "Misconduct" is any conviction of an offence under the Criminal Code of Canada unless, in the opinion of the disciplinary committee, the offence had no relation to the veterinarian's qualifications to practise.

Legislated rules of ethics are contained in the bylaws of the Prince Edward Island Veterinary Medical Association. The preamble to the code reads as follows:

> The honour and dignity of the Veterinary Medical profession lies in its obedience to a just and reasonable code of ethics set forth herein as a guide to its members. The object of this code, however, is more far-reaching, for exemplary professional conduct not only upholds honour and dignity, but also enlarges our sphere of usefulness, exalts our social standards and promotes the science we cultivate. Briefly stated, our "Code of Professional Ethics" is the foundation of the individual and collective efforts of veterinarians. It is based upon the Golden Rule.

The preamble is then followed by guidelines, which specify that the veterinarian "should first of all be a good citizen and a leader in movements to advance community welfare." The "golden rule" approach of Newfoundland and Labrador and Prince Edward Island is also espoused in the preamble to the bylaws of the Nova Scotia Veterinary Medical Association.

Similarly, the bylaws of the Saskatchewan Veterinary Medical Association contain a statutory code of ethics that addresses responsibilities to the client, responsibilities to the profession, and responsibilities to society generally. Among the "responsibilities to the client" are a prohibition on guaranteeing any cure and a requirement that the veterinarian know his or her limitations and when necessary refer the client to other opinions and services. Like the Prince Edward Island bylaws, the Saskatchewan bylaws make reference to the responsibility of the practitioner to "educate himself and to adjust to modern concepts of veterinary medicine in order to ensure the best possible service to his clients and patients." The Saskatchewan practitioner is required to attend at least ten hours of continuing education classes per year. Under the heading "responsibilities to the profession," the code specifies the type and amount of acceptable advertising. A helpful provision describes advertising that is "considered objectionable," including that which promotes personal superiority over another, secret remedies, or advertising as a corporation or partnership. Members of the profession are prohibited from belittling or injuring the professional standing of another. General compliance with federal, provincial, and municipal law is required as the hallmark of one's responsibilities to society as a whole.

A well-organized code of ethics appears in appendix A to the bylaws of the British Columbia Veterinary Medical Association. Under headings such as "General Deportment," which requires exemplary personal conduct, and "Professional Deportment," which requires courtesy and respect to fellow members, the British Columbia code has as its objective the desire to maintain the integrity of the profession while protecting the public.

ADVERTISING

As mentioned in chapter 4, the provincial laws that regulate the profession often set out limitations on advertising the services of a veterinary practice. In some cases, these matters are dealt with in the statutory codes of ethics referred to above, on the ground that advertising is a matter of ethical practice as opposed to a practice management issue.

In Newfoundland and Labrador, the bylaws of the Veterinary Medical Association set out guidelines relating to advertising. While advertising is not prohibited outright, the bylaws state that advertising as a means of obtaining patronage is objectionable in the practice of any branch of veterinary medicine. It is denounced as unethical and unprofessional. This suggests that any form of promotional advertising is prohibited in Newfoundland and Labrador except for directory advertisements, local newspapers, business cards and letterhead, and some display signs, all of which are specifically addressed in the bylaws. For instance, local newspaper ads are customary and advisable but they must be "reasonable" in size and display and should be limited to the name, title, address, office hours, and telephone number of the practice.

The rules in Prince Edward Island are similar to the Newfoundland and Ontario rules relating to advertising. A general prohibition on advertising for the purpose of soliciting patronage or professional services is set out, followed by exemptions for communicating with "regular clients" so long as such documents are marked "advertisement." The letterhead of a member of the Prince Edward Island Association must be "modest, announcing at most, name, title, address, telephone numbers, office hours and a preference for a specified species."

Among the most comprehensive guidelines for veterinary advertising, the bylaws of the Nova Scotia Veterinary Medical Association are specific concerning the types and display of advertising. Once again, there is a general prohibition on advertising for the sake of "obtaining patronage." However, guidelines for "acceptable advertising" are set out, which include writing articles for the local press to announce the presence of contagious diseases, provided that the writer's bona fide intention is to "salvage the livestock of clients rather than personal gain." Client reminders are also permitted. Separate rules are set out for telephone directory advertising, including a limitation on the size of an ad. Business cards may be distributed only to clients, colleagues, and business and academic contacts, and a card can be printed only on paper; it cannot be magnetized or manufactured in such a way that it can be attached to anything else, and it cannot exceed a specified size.

In Nova Scotia, newspaper advertising is similarly regulated, and can be used only to announce a new facility, a change of location, a change in ownership, a change in phone number or office hours, or a new associate, or in cases where a telephone directory ad has not yet appeared. In each case the number and frequency of ads are restricted. Exterior signage is restricted to sixty square feet on one side; a sign may be illuminated continuously but not intermittently. The sign may include the name of the hospital, the name of the individuals practising there, the telephone number, and the international symbol for veterinary medicine. No other logos, drawings, or pictures may be included on an exterior sign. The regulations in Nova Scotia even go into some detail about what is permitted in a client information letter. Veterinarians are prohibited from publishing any letter that, in the opinion of the council of the association, is self-serving or self-gratifying, indicates fees or discounted services, or contains any comparison of any of the services of any other veterinary facility.

Bylaw 20 of the New Brunswick Veterinary Medical Association sets out detailed rules for advertising similar to those contained in the regulations to the Ontario Veterinarians Act. Among other things, the New Brunswick legislation imposes a general prohibition on advertising except as permitted by the bylaw. Bylaw 20.03 allows the veterinarian to communicate "factual, accurate and verifiable" information that a reasonable person would consider relevant in the choice of a veterinarian. Such materials cannot contain false or misleading statements, must be dignified and in good taste, must not contain any testimonials or information relating to fees to be charged, and must make no reference to a specific drug, appliance, or equipment. Fee schedules can be displayed in the veterinary facility, provided that the size and location of the schedule is such that a person looking in from the outside cannot read it. The steering of clients to a particular veterinary practice is prohibited, as is the solicitation of clients. However, a veterinarian may send written communications to persons who generally might find such information useful, or distribute general or preventive health care information to regular clients. Reminder notices are permitted. (Regular clients are defined as persons who regularly use the services of a member with reasonable frequency and who have not requested that records be forwarded to another veterinarian.) The restriction against steering does not apply to a professional referral from one practitioner to another.

In addition to setting out detailed guidelines relating to veterinary advertising, the Alberta regulations address the issue of advertisements for "non-veterinary medical business," which includes any business activity that is not veterinary medicine as defined in the Alberta Veterinary Profession Act. Such non-veterinary advertising is prohibited, except if the other business has a separate phone number that is not used in the veterinary practice. The names of the two businesses cannot resemble each other, and the word "veterinary" or "veterinarian" cannot be employed in any manner or symbol.

The Alberta Veterinary Medical Association has published guidelines on advertising in professional directories. In what appears to be candid support for advertising, the Alberta regulatory body indicates that it "supports the right of practitioners to list and identify their practice in directories available to the public in a given geographical area." The guidelines specify those items that may be listed in the directory. Anything not directly referred to must be submitted to the association's council for approval.

The British Columbia statutory code of ethics deals with advertising as part of any marketing activity and, like the codes of the other provinces, requires such activity to be true and objective, accurate and verifiable, not capable of misleading, and not in "bad taste, offensive, self-laudatory, or otherwise contrary to the honour and dignity of the veterinary profession." The onus is on the practitioner to ensure that these requirements are met.

In Quebec, advertising is governed by regulations passed under the Professional Code. Section 5 of the advertising regulation sets out the information that may be contained in advertisements, including the practitioner's name, degree, address, and telephone number, and the graphic symbol of the profession.

The issue of the timing of telephone directory advertising was reviewed by the British Columbia Supreme Court in *Bond v. British Columbia Veterinary Medical Association* (31 CPR (3d) 499) in 1990. A veterinarian was said to have engaged in professional misconduct when the name of his clinic was advertised in the telephone directory before the name was approved by the association. The veterinarian said that he thought the telephone company representative had told him that the listing could be cancelled until October, when in fact it could only be cancelled until June. The name to be approved was "Spay and Neuter Clinic," which was later rejected by the association as denoting a specialty. The veterinarian was found guilty of professional misconduct and fined $10,000. The veterinarian was successful in the later application for judicial review; the court held that the refusal to approve the name was to be reconsidered by the association since in the court's opinion the name was merely suggestive of procedures that fell within a general practice. The finding of professional misconduct was set aside.

One might ask whether these restrictions in provincial legislation offend the Canadian Charter of Rights and Freedoms as an unreasonable restriction on freedom of expression. This is the essence of an Ontario case, *Jafine and Catherwood v. College of Veterinarians of Ontario* (5 OR (3d) 439) which is as yet undecided. In 1991 the case was brought to the Divisional Court of Ontario for the purpose of prohibiting proceedings before the discipline committee. Two veterinarians were charged with professional misconduct in connection with advertisements published by them. Among other things, the ads contained statements such as "The best pet care you'll find anywhere" and "we can take care of ALL your pet's health needs under one roof." The discipline committee of the College of Veterinarians of Ontario found these advertisements objectionable in that they were not verifiable and could be misleading to the public. A reference to a "Free Pet Exam" was viewed by the discipline committee as a form of price advertising in contravention of the Veterinarians Act of Ontario. The principal issue to be determined was whether the restrictions on advertising contravened the Canadian Charter of Rights and Freedoms' guarantee of freedom of expression, which includes freedom of the press and other media of communication. The Supreme Court of Canada addressed this issue in *Royal College of Dental Surgeons v. Rocket* ([1990] 2 SCR) in 1990:

> It is difficult to overstate the importance in our society of proper regulation of our learned professions. Indeed, it is not disputed that the provinces have a legitimate interest in regulating professional advertising. The maintenance of professionalism and the protection of the public are at the heart of such regulations. If a dentist or other professional claims to be more competent than his or her colleagues, there is no way in which an average consumer can verify that claim. In such circumstances professional regulation of advertising is clearly justified.

The discipline committee asserted that while the restrictions did breach the Charter of Rights and Freedoms, the restriction constituted a reasonable limitation as provided for in the Charter.

Section 60.1 of the Professional Code of Quebec states that any service provided by the veterinarian must conform with the statements he or she makes or any advertisement he or she places. The veterinarian is prohibited from making any false or misleading statement, in particular as to his or her level of competence or the scope of his or her effectiveness.

CONTINUING EDUCATION

Practitioners are obliged to maintain their levels of competence so as to discharge their legal liability to clients and avoid negligence claims; but they are also under an ethical obligation to maintain their competence through continuing education.

Section 18 of the bylaws of the Prince Edward Island Veterinary Medical Association states that every holder of a licence in that province has a requirement in every two-year calendar period to attend and participate in not less than twenty hours of continuing education courses in veterinary medicine. Those courses must be approved by the council of the association. Failure to attend and to notify the registrar of attendance can result in suspension.   Continuing education is addressed in Quebec by regulations passed under the Professional Code and the Veterinary Surgeons Act. In the event that the Bureau is of the opinion that a member's level of competence falls short of the requirements for the protection of the public, it can require the practitioner to undertake a training period, which may consist of practical training, studies, courses, or research work.

Continuing education is required under the general regulations to the Veterinary Profession Act in Alberta. The bylaws were amended in January 1993 to include provisions dictating that active members of the Alberta Veterinary Medical Association must accumulate at least ten credit hours of mandatory continuing education per year. Evidence of having completed such courses is by way of a certificate presented by the member at the time of renewing his or her registration. The Alberta provisions specify that one credit hour must consist of a scientific lecture and/or wet lab sponsored by an international, national, provincial, or state veterinary organization or an approved local veterinary group.

AUTHORITY TO PRACTISE

In Prince Edward Island, it is a breach of professional ethics for any veterinarian to intentionally place his or her professional knowledge or services at the disposal of any group or individual for the purpose of encouraging unqualified persons to diagnose and prescribe for the ailments and diseases of animals. Under section 24.2.6 of the bylaws of the Veterinary Medical Association, such conduct is especially reprehensible when it is done to promote commercial interest and monetary gain. Thus the profession itself charges its members with ensuring that no unauthorized practising of veterinary medicine takes place, as "such deportment is beneath the dignity of professional ethics and practice; it can be harmful to both the welfare of the animal-owning public and the veterinary profession; it violates principles of humane animal care; it may cause great economic loss and endanger public health and is, therefore, contrary to sound public policy."

In British Columbia, the code of ethics addresses the relationship between the veterinarian and the pharmacist. While licensed pharmacists are to be recognized by members of the veterinary profession and their services used, the veterinarian is under a duty not to provide such recognition or use such services if the pharmacist purports to diagnose and prescribe treatments for sick animals. Such conduct is to be viewed as prejudicial to the public interest, contrary to the laws governing veterinary medical practice, and in violation of provincial and federal laws enacted for the control of animal diseases.

The Veterinary Profession Act of the Northwest Territories defines "veterinary surgery" to include the surgical, dental, and medical treatment of animals; however, the legislation specifically provides that certain procedures such as castration, spaying, vaccinating, and dehorning is not within the definition. Thus it appears that lay persons can, without challenge, perform those procedures; in a remote jurisdiction, where veterinarians may not be nearby, these exclusions make sense. In addition, in the Northwest Territories, any person who practises veterinary medicine without the appropriate licence or who uses the title "veterinary surgeon" or any abbreviation thereof in his or her name can be charged with a quasi-criminal offence and, upon conviction, subject to nominal fines. Any such prosecution must be commenced within one year from the time at which the alleged offence arose.

REPORTING MISTREATMENT

The Quebec code of ethics for veterinarians contains a unique provision, which specifies that the veterinary surgeon is under an ethical obligation to report to appropriate animal protection authorities any mistreatment of an animal. Even in the absence of any provincial requirement to report mistreatment, the veterinarian has a moral obligation to deal with mistreatment in the light of the provisions of the Veterinarian's Oath.

CONFLICT OF INTEREST

The Veterinarians Act of Ontario provides that continuing to practise in a situation where a conflict of interest is evident is deemed to be professional misconduct, which can give rise to disciplinary proceedings. A conflict of interest arises when certain actions involve a "related person" of the veterinarian, which is, generally, anyone with whom the veterinarian is connected by blood, marriage, or adoption. A veterinarian has a conflict of interest if he or she, or a related person, or an employee or employer of the veterinarian enters into any agreement, including a lease of premises, under which any amount payable by or to the veterinarian or a related person is connected to the fees charged by the veterinarian. A conflict also arises if the agreement makes or confers a fee, credit, or other benefit by reason of a referral from or to any person. The general exception to these types of agreements is a partnership agreement with another veterinarian, whereby the draws of the partners or other partnership interests are tied directly to the amount billed by the respective partners.

A conflict also arises if a veterinarian assesses an animal on behalf of both the vendor and the purchaser of the animal or if the practitioner is regularly engaged by either the vendor or the purchaser and inspects the animal of behalf of the other party in the transaction. A conflict will not arise if the assessment is carried out for both parties; that is, if they both consent to the engagement before the examination is conducted and after they are informed of the conflict that would otherwise arise. The clear obligation on the veterinarian in these cases is to ensure that both parties recognize that any information obtained by the veterinarian cannot be maintained confidentially and kept from the other party.

The bylaws of the Veterinary Medical Association of Newfoundland and Labrador provide that "when employed by a buyer to inspect an animal for soundness, it is unacceptable [for the veterinarian] to accept a fee from the seller. The acceptance of such a fee is prima facie evidence of fraud." Conflict of interest rules are set out in the Prince Edward Island legislation relating to pre-purchase inspections conducted by a veterinarian. It is evidence of fraud if the practitioner accepts a fee from the seller when he or she is also engaged by the purchaser. Practitioners in Prince Edward Island are subject to conflict of interest rules when they enter into an agreement, including a lease of premises, under which any amount payable by the veterinarian or a related person is related to the fees charged by the veterinarian.

MAKING AFTER-HOURS SERVICES AVAILABLE

The regulations and bylaws under provincial veterinary legislation state that all veterinarians in private practice are responsible for providing reasonably prompt services outside regular hours if the services are medically necessary for animals that the veterinarian has recently treated or that the veterinarian treats regularly. This ethical obligation can be discharged by referring the client to another veterinarian who has agreed to cover your practice for a period or to an emergency clinic, provided that you are responsible for promptly continuing the treatment after the animal is discharged from the emergency clinic until the treatment is no longer necessary or until the client has a reasonable opportunity to engage the services of another veterinarian.

APPENDIX A

THIS INDENTURE made the 15th day of February, 1994.

IN PURSUANCE OF THE SHORT FORM OF LEASES ACT:

B E T W E E N :

<u>ABC RENTAL CORPORATION</u>
(hereinafter called the "Lessor")

OF THE FIRST PART

- and -

<u>DR. JOHN WHITE</u>
(hereinafter called the "Lessee")

OF THE SECOND PART

WITNESSETH that in consideration of the rents, covenants and agreements hereinafter reserved and contained on the part of the said Lessee, to be paid, observed and performed, the said Lessor has demised and leased and by these presents doth demise and lease unto the said Lessee.

ALL THOSE CERTAIN PREMISES excluding any part of the external walls known and described as part of Lot 12, Registered Plan 123, in the Town of Anywhere, County of Anyplace and municipally known as 123 Main Street.

TERM

TO HAVE AND TO HOLD the demised premises for and during the term of Five (5) years, to be computed from the 1st day of March, 1994, and from thenceforth ensuing and to be fully completed and ended upon the 28th day of February, 1999.

RENTAL

YIELDING AND PAYING therefor yearly and every year during the said term hereby granted, unto the said Lessor, the sum of Twenty-four Thousand ($24,000.00) Dollars per annum, payable in equal monthly instalments of Two Thousand ($2,000.00) Dollars each in advance on the 1st day of each and every month during the said term, the first payment to be made on the 1st day of March, 1994, which said payment is exclusive of any tax, levy or charge required by the Goods and Services Tax Act (Canada) or other legislation; the Lessee hereby acknowledging that he shall pay to the Lessor all such taxes, levies or charges in addition to the rental set out herein.

THE SAID LESSEE covenants with the said Lessor to pay rent;

BUSINESS TAXES

AND to pay all business taxes and BIA assessments in respect of the business carried on by the Lessee in and upon or by reason of their occupancy of the premises hereby demised;

REPAIRS

AND to repair (reasonable wear and tear and damage by fire, lightning and tempest only excepted);

AND that the said Lessor may enter and view state of repair;

AND that the said Lessee will repair according to notice in writing (reasonable wear and tear and damage by fire, lightning and tempest excepted);

AND that they will leave the premises in good repair (reasonable wear and tear and damage by fire, lightning and tempest only excepted);

ASSIGNMENT

AND will not assign or sublet the whole or any part of the demised premises without leave; the Lessee hereby waives and renounces the benefit of any present or future act of the Legislature of Ontario which would allow the Lessee to assign or sublet this lease, without leave of the Lessor.

AND THE SAID LESSEE covenants with the said Lessor, its successors and assigns:

TYPE OF BUSINESS

(a)   **THAT** the said demised premises will not, during the said term, be at any time used for any other purpose than that of a professional veterinary hospital together with the sale of ancillary products and services.

FIXTURES

(b)   **THAT** no fixtures, goods or chattels of any kind will, except in the ordinary course of business, be removed from the demised premises during the term hereby demised or at any time thereafter without the written consent of the Lessor, its successors or assigns, being first had and obtained, until all rent in arrears as well as all rent to become due during the remainder of the term hereby granted shall have been fully paid, or the payment thereof secured to the satisfaction of the Lessor or its assigns.

ELECTRIC POWER

(c)   **THAT** the Lessee will not, during the said term or at any time prior or subsequent thereto, purchase, acquire or use any electric current for lighting or other purposes except from the company or corporation which shall for the time supply the Lessor with electric current for such purposes in the said building; the intention being that without the written consent of the Lessor, there shall be only one system of electric lighting in the said building.

(d) **THE** Lessee hereby covenants to pay all charges for electric energy (for light and power) and gas used by the Lessee in the demised premises.

PARTITIONS, ALTERATIONS

(e) **THAT** if the Lessee shall, during the said term, desire to affix or erect partitions, counters or fixtures in any part of the walls, floors or ceilings of the demised premises, it may do so at its own expense at any time and from time to time provided that the Lessee's rights to make such alterations to the demised premises shall be subject to the following conditions:

(1) **THAT** before undertaking any such alterations, the Lessee shall submit to the Lessor a plan showing the proposed alterations and shall obtain the approval and consent of the Lessor to the same.

(2) **THAT** all such alterations shall conform to all building by-laws, if any, then in force affecting the demised premises.

(3) **THAT** such alterations will not be of such kind or extent as to in any manner weaken the structure of the building after the alterations are completed or reduce the value of the building.

(f) **THAT**, except as herein provided, the Lessee will not erect or affix or remove or change the location or style of any partitions or fixtures, without the written consent of the Lessor being first had and obtained.

(g) **THAT**, at the expiration of the term hereby granted, or any renewal thereof, all fixtures belonging to the Lessee shall remain upon the demised premises until taken down by the Lessor, and the Lessee shall forthwith, upon the same being taken down, remove the same from the demised premises first paying to the Lessor the expense of such taking down and making good all damage occasioned to the demised premises by the taking down or removal thereof.

BANKRUPTCY OR INSOLVENCY

(h)   **THAT**, if the term hereby granted or the goods and chattels of the Lessee or any assignee or subtenant shall be at any time seized or taken in execution or attachment, or if the Lessee or any such assignee or subtenant shall make an assignment for the benefit of creditors or shall become bankrupt or insolvent, or make a proposal to its creditors, or without the consent of the Lessor being first obtained in writing, shall make a sale under the Bulk Sales Act in respect of goods on the premises, or being a company shall become subject to any legislative enactment relating to liquidation or winding up, either voluntary or compulsory, the said term shall immediately become forfeited and void and an amount equivalent to the next ensuing three months' rent shall be at once due and payable.

RULES AND REGULATIONS

(i)   **THAT** the Lessee and its clerks, servants and agents will at all times during the occupancy of the demised premises observe and conform to such reasonable rules and regulations as shall be made by the Lessor from time to time and of which the Lessee shall be notified, such rules and regulations being deemed to be incorporated in and form part of these presents.

EXPROPRIATION OR CONDEMNATION

(j)   **IT IS AGREED** between the Parties hereto that if the said premises be expropriated or condemned by any department of the federal, provincial or municipal government then the Lessor shall have the right, notwithstanding anything herein contained, to terminate this lease upon giving three months' notice in writing to the Lessee of his intention so to do or by paying the said Lessee a bonus of three months' rent, in which latter event, the Lessee undertakes to vacate the said premises at the expiration of thirty (30) days from the delivery of such notice.

PROTECTIVE INSTALLATIONS

(k) **THE LESSEE** agrees to pay the cost of any installations, additions, or alterations to the said premises that the Lessor may be required to make by any municipal, provincial or other governing authority, or requested by any private protective system used by the Lessee, for the security and protection of the Lessee and his employees and his or their effects including, but not so as to limit the foregoing installations, additions and alterations for fire and theft protection, and all such installations, additions, or alterations shall forthwith become the property of the Lessor.

DISTRESS

(l) **AND** the Lessee further covenants, promises and agrees with the Lessor that notwithstanding any present or future Act of the Legislature of the Province of Ontario, none of the goods or chattels of the Lessee at any time during the continuance of the term hereby created on the said demised premises shall be exempt from levy by distress for rent in arrears by the Lessee as provided for by the said section of said Act, and that upon any claim being made for such exemption by the Lessee or on distress being made by the Lessor, this covenant and agreement may be pleaded as an estoppel against the Lessee in any action brought to test the right to the levying upon any such goods as are named exempted in the said section, the Lessee waiving as he hereby does all and every benefit that could or might have accrued to him under and by virtue of the said section of the said Act but for the above covenant.

THE LESSOR COVENANTS with the Lessee for quiet enjoyment.

THE LESSOR FURTHER COVENANTS with the Lessee as follows:

TAXES AND RATES

(a) **TO** pay all taxes and rates, municipal, parliamentary or otherwise, including water rates for the normal supply of cold water to the said premises, assessed against the demised premises of the Lessor or

Lessee on account thereof, saving and excepting any business taxes and taxes upon personal property or income of the Lessee, licence fees, or other taxes imposed upon the property, business or income of the Lessee;

PROVIDED THAT;

(i)   **IN THE EVENT** of the Lessee being assessed as a separate school supporter, and by reason thereof the amount of the taxes payable on the said premises being increased over the amount payable on an assessment as a public school supporter, then and in such event the Lessee covenants and agrees with the Lessor to pay to the Lessor the amount of such increase upon demand being made therefor in writing by the Lessor. It is understood and agreed that such increase shall be payable by the Lessee notwithstanding the fact that at the time such demand is made, the Lessee may have ceased to be a tenant of the Lessor. In the event of the Lessee failing to pay to the Lessor the amount of such increase upon demand as herein provided, then the Lessor shall have the same rights and remedies for collection thereof as for the rent in arrears.

(ii)   **THE LESSEE** covenants and agrees to and with the Lessor that if there shall be an increase in municipal taxes payable by the Lessor over the amount shown by the immediately last tax bill issued by the municipality in which the demised premises are situate prior to the date of this lease, the Lessee will pay any such increase apportioned over the term of the within lease and the renewal (if any) hereinbefore provided and that any such increase in municipal taxes shall be deemed to be part of the rent reserved hereunder and all the remedies available to the Lessor relating to rent both hereunder and at law shall apply, mutatis mutandis, thereto.

HEATING

(b)   **TO** heat the said premises between the 15th day of October and the 1st day of May next ensuing in each year in such manner as to keep the said premises at a reasonable temperature for the reasonable use thereof by the Lessee during reasonable business hours, except during the making of repairs, and in case the boilers, engines, pipes, or other apparatus or any of them used in effecting the heating of the said demised premises shall at any time become incapable of heating said premises as aforesaid, or be damaged or destroyed, to repair said damage or replace said boilers, engines, pipes or apparatus or any of them or (at the option of the Lessor) substitute other heating apparatus therefor within a reasonable time; provided, however, that the Lessor shall not be liable for indirect or consequential damages for personal discomfort or illness arising from any default of the Lessor.

ACCESS

(c)   **TO** give the Lessee, his agents, clerks, servants and all persons transacting business with the Lessee, in common with other persons, the right to enter the demised premises by means of the main entrance at all reasonable times, subject to rules and regulations in regard to the said building as may be passed from time to time.

PROVISO for re-entry by the said Lessor on non-payment of rent or non-performance of covenants.

VOIDANCE OF LEASE VACANT OR IMPROPER USE

IT IS FURTHER DECLARED AND AGREED that in case the said premises or any part thereof become and remain vacant and unoccupied for the period of fifteen (15) days, or be used by any other person or persons, or for any other purpose than as above provided, without the written consent of the Lessor, this lease shall, at the option of the Lessor, cease and be void and the term hereby created expire and be at an end, anything hereinbefore to the contrary notwithstanding and the proportionate part of the current rent shall thereupon become immediately due and payable, and the Lessor may re-enter and take possession of the premises as though the Lessee or other occupant or occupants of said premises were holding over after the expiration of the term; or in such case instead of determining this lease as aforesaid and re-entering upon the demised premises, the Lessor may take possession of the demised premises, or any part or parts thereof, and let and manage the same and grant any lease or leases thereof upon such terms as to the Lessor or its assigns may appear to be reasonable, and demand, collect, receive and distrain for all rental which shall become payable in respect thereof, and apply the said rentals after deducting all expenses incurred in connection with the demised premises and in the collection of the said rent including reasonable commission for the collection thereof and the management of the demised premises, upon the rent hereby reserved, and the Lessor and its assigns and every such agent acting as aforesaid from time to time, shall in so acting be the agents of the Lessee, who alone shall be responsible for their acts, and the Lessor and its assigns shall not be accountable for any moneys except those actually received, notwithstanding any act, neglect, omission or default of any such agent acting as aforesaid.

WATER AND GAS DAMAGE

AND IT IS FURTHER DECLARED AND AGREED THAT the Lessor shall not be liable for any damage to any property at any time upon the demised premises arising from gas, steam, water, rain or snow which may leak into, issue or flow from any part of the said building, or from the gas, water, steam or drainage pipes or plumbing works of the same or from any other place or quarter or for any damage caused by or attributable to the condition or arrangement of any electric or other wires in the said building.

The Lessee shall be liable for any damage done by reason of water being left running from the taps in the demised premises or from gas permitted to escape therein.

RISKS OF INJURY

AND the Lessor shall not be responsible for any personal injury which shall be sustained by the Lessee or any employee, customer, or other person who may be upon the demised premises or in the said building or the entrances or appurtenances thereto. All risks of any such injury being assumed by the Lessee, who shall hold the Lessor harmless and indemnified therefrom.

NOTICE OF ACCIDENT

THE Lessee shall give the Lessor prompt written notice of any accident or other defect in the sprinkler system, water pipes, gas pipes or heating apparatus, telephone, electric or other wires on any part of the premises.

INSURANCE

THE Lessee covenants with the said Lessor that his said business to be so carried on in the said building will not be of such a nature as to increase the insurance risk on the said premises or cause the Lessor to pay an increased rate of insurance premiums on the said premises by reason thereof and it is distinctly understood that in case said business so carried on by the Lessee is or becomes of such a nature to increase the insurance risk or causes the Lessor and/or other occupants of the said building to pay an increased rate of insurance premiums, that the Lessee will from time to time pay to the Lessor the increased amount of insurance premiums which the said Lessor and other occupants of the said building have to pay in consequence thereof; provided that the Lessee covenants that he will not carry on or permit to be carried on any business in the said building which may make void or voidable any insurance held by the Lessor or the other occupants of the said building.

BUSINESS NOT TO BE A NUISANCE

PROVIDED that the Lessee will not do or permit anything to be done on the said premises or permit or keep anything therein which may be annoying to the Lessor or other occupants of the said building or which the said Lessor may deem to be a nuisance and that no machinery shall be used therein which shall cause any undue vibration in or to the said premises and that in case of the Lessor or any other occupants of the said building reasonably complaining that any machinery or operation or process is a nuisance to it or them or which causes any undue vibration or noise in the said premises, that upon receiving notice thereof, the said Lessee will immediately abate such nuisance. The said Lessee covenants not to obstruct or interfere with the rights of the Lessor or other occupants of the said building or in any way injure or annoy them or conflict with any of the rules and regulations of the Board of Health or with any statute or municipal bylaw.

SIGN

AND IT IS HEREBY FURTHER AGREED by and between the said Lessor and the said Lessee that no sign, advertisement or notice shall be inscribed, painted or affixed by the said Lessee on any part of the outside or inside of the building whatever, unless of such manner, colour, size and style and in such places upon or in said building as shall be first designated by the Lessor, and, furthermore, the Lessee, on ceasing to be lessee of the demised premises, will, before removing his goods and fixtures from the said premises, cause any sign as aforesaid to be removed or obliterated at his own expense and in a workmanlike manner to the satisfaction of the Lessor.

ELEVATOR

THE Lessor undertakes to maintain elevators in the said building which are to be run during the ordinary business hours of every business day of the year, but not during public holidays or Sundays, except at the option of the Lessor. The Lessee shall, subject to the Lessor's rules and regulations, have free use of such elevators in common with others lawfully using the same, but the Lessee and his employees and all other persons using any such elevator shall do so at his, her or their sole risk, and under no circumstances shall the Lessor be held responsible for any damage or injury happening to any person whilst using such elevator, or occasioned to any person by such elevator or any appurtenances and whether such damage or injury shall happen by reason of the act, omission or negligence or otherwise of the Lessor, or any of its employees, servants, agents or otherwise howsoever.

WATER

THE Lessor agrees to pay for normal water consumed on the said premises, but in the event of any abnormal consumption of water either by reason of the character of the business carried on by the Lessee or by the use of mechanical or other contrivances, the Lessee consents to the installation of a water meter at his own expense, if necessary, and further agrees to pay for the excess water consumed on the said premises.

PLATE GLASS

THE Lessee agrees, at his own expense, to replace any plate glass or other glass that has been broken or removed during the term of the within lease or of any renewal thereof and will during the said term keep the plate glass fully insured in some company approved by the Lessor.

___

FIRE

PROVIDED THAT, if during the term herein or any renewal thereof, the premises shall be destroyed or damaged by fire or the elements, then the following provisions shall apply:

(a)   If the demised premises shall be so badly injured as to be unfit for occupancy, and as to be incapable of being repaired with reasonable diligence within one hundred and twenty (120) days of the happening of such injury, then the term hereby granted shall cease and be at an end to all intents and purposes from the date of such damage or destruction, and the Lessee shall immediately surrender the same and yield up possession of the demised premises to the Lessor, and the rent from the time of such surrender shall be apportioned;

(b)   If the demised premises shall be capable, with reasonable diligence, of being repaired and rendered fit for occupancy within one hundred and twenty (120) days from the happening of such injury as aforesaid, but if the damage is such as to render the demised premises wholly unfit for occupancy, then the rent hereby reserved shall not run or accrue after such injury, or while the process of repair is going on, and the Lessor shall repair the same with all reasonable speed, and the rent shall recommence immediately after such repairs shall be completed;

(c)   If the demised premises shall be repaired within one hundred and twenty (120) days as aforesaid and if the damage is such that the said premises are capable of being partially used, then until such damage shall have been repaired, the rent shall abate in the proportion that the part of the demised premises rendered unfit for occupancy bears to the whole of the demised premises.

NO ABATEMENT OF RENT

THERE shall be no abatement from or reduction of the rent due hereunder, nor shall the Lessee be entitled to damages, losses, costs or disbursements from the Lessor during the term hereby created on, caused by or on account of fire, (except as above), water, sprinkler systems, partial or temporary failure or stoppage of heat, light, elevator, live steam or plumbing service in or to the said premises or building, whether due to acts of God, strikes, accidents, the making of alterations, repairs, renewals, improvements, structural changes to the said premises or buildings or the equipment or systems supplying the said services, or from any cause whatsoever; provided that the said failure or stoppage be remedied within a reasonable time.

RIGHT TO SHOW PREMISES

THAT the Lessee will permit the Lessor to exhibit the demised premises during the last three (3) months of the term to any prospective tenant and will permit all persons having written authority therefor to view the said premises at all reasonable hours.

NOTICES

THAT any notice which either of the parties is required or permitted to give pursuant to any provision of this lease may, if intended for the Lessee, be given by a writing left at the demised premises or mailed by registered mail addressed to the Lessee at the demised premises, and if intended for the Lessor by a writing left at the premises of the Lessor or mailed by registered mail addressed to the Lessor at the Lessor's said premises, and such notice shall be deemed to have been given at the time it was delivered or mailed, as the case may be.

OVER HOLDING

PROVIDED FURTHER, and it is hereby agreed, that should the Lessee hold over after the expiration of this lease and the Lessor thereafter accepts rent for the said premises, the Lessee shall hold the said premises as a monthly tenant only of the Lessor but subject in all other respects to the terms and conditions of this lease.

The words importing the singular number only shall include the plural, and vice versa, and words importing the masculine gender shall include the feminine gender, and words importing persons shall include firms and corporations and vice versa.

Unless the context otherwise required, the word "Lessor" and the word "Lessee" wherever used herein shall be construed to include and shall mean the executors, administrators, successors and/or assigns of the said Lessor and Lessee, respectively, and when there are two or more Lessees bound by the same covenants herein contained, their obligations shall be joint and several.

IN WITNESS WHEREOF the parties hereto have executed these presents.

SIGNED, SEALED
AND DELIVERED

in the presence of

_____
John White, DVM

ABC Rental Corporation

per.   _____
Joe Doe, President

APPENDIX B

Asset Purchase Agreement

OFFER TO PURCHASE

(Under The Bulk Sales Act)

I, JOHN WHITE,

of the Town of Anywhere, in the County of Anyplace   **(as Purchaser)**,

HEREBY AGREE TO AND WITH

JANE BLACK,

of the City of Anyville, in the Regional Municipality

of Anycounty   **(as Vendor)**

to purchase the assets described below on the terms set forth in this Agreement:

1.00   Assets Purchased

1.01   All the assets including the goodwill, trade name, leasehold interest, goods, professional veterinary equipment, client and patient lists, accounts receivable, all medical records, chattels, fixtures, stock-in-trade, inventory and contents of the professional veterinary practice known as "Fantasy Veterinary Clinic" and situated at 123 Main Street, Anyville, Ontario (the

"Practice"), as now located upon the said premises and inspected and approved by the Purchaser. See Schedule "A" attached for the list of equipment and fixtures included in the purchase price.

2.00 Purchase Price

2.01 The purchase price shall be THREE HUNDRED AND FIFTY THOUSAND ($350,000.00) DOLLARS inclusive of the value of all stock-in-trade and inventory. The total of the said sums being herein referred to as the aggregate purchase price.

2.02 The aggregate purchase price shall be payable as follows:

(a) A deposit of ONE THOUSAND ($1,000.00) DOLLARS by cash or certified cheque to the said Vendor on this date to be held in trust pending completion or other termination of this Agreement, and to be credited on account of purchase money on closing;

(b) by the issuance and delivery by the Purchaser to the Vendor of a Promissory Note in the principal amount of THREE HUNDRED THOUSAND ($300,000.00) DOLLARS together with interest thereon at the rate of EIGHT PER CENT (8%) per annum and repayable in equal monthly blended payments of FOUR THOUSAND FIVE HUNDRED ($4,500.00) DOLLARS, with each such payment to be credited first to interest and the balance of each such payment applied to principal, and payable on the 1st day of each month commencing on the 1st day of August, 1994 through to and including the 1st day of July, 2004 which Promissory Note shall contain a privilege in favour of the Purchaser permitting the prepayment of all or any portion of the principal outstanding from time to time without notice, penalty or bonus; and

(c) the balance of the purchase price shall be payable on closing subject to adjustments.

2.03   This offer shall be conditional until the 15th day of July, 1994 upon the Purchaser arranging satisfactory financing to complete the within transaction failing which this offer shall be null and void and of no further force and effect and the deposit returned to the Purchaser without interest or deduction. This condition is inserted for the sole benefit of the Purchaser and may be waived by him at any time prior to its expiry.

3.00   Allocation of Purchase Price

3.01   The purchase price herein shall be allocated among the assets purchased hereunder as follows:

Goodwill	$300,000.00
Leasehold interest, equipment and other assets	47,000.00
Inventory	3,000.00
TOTAL	$350,000.00

4.00   Excluded Assets

4.01   It is agreed that there shall be specifically excluded from the purchase and sale herein, the following:

(a) Cash-on-hand or in a bank or other depositories; and

(b) books of account of the Vendor excluding customer lists and any operating records.

5.00   Adjustments

5.01   Taxes, rents, water, gas and hydro rates and insurance and other similar or usual prepaid expenses relating to the Practice and assets hereby agreed to be purchased and sold, shall be adjusted as of the date of closing.

6.00   Date of Closing

6.01   The sale shall be completed on the 31st day of July, 1994, on which date possession of the Practice and assets above described is to be given to the Purchaser.

7.00   Lease

7.01 (a) The Vendor represents and warrants that there is a good, valid and subsisting lease of the premises known as 123 Main Street, Anyville, Ontario for a term of five (5) years expiring on the 30th day of October, 1994, at a monthly rental of $1,700.00 and it is a condition of this Offer that the Vendor obtain the written consent of the Lessor to the assignment of the said lease to the Purchaser within ten (10) days of the date of acceptance, failing which this Offer shall be null and void and the deposit returned in full without interest.

(b) Notwithstanding the generality of the foregoing, it shall be a condition of this Offer that the Vendor obtain the written consent of the Lessor to amend the lease referred to in subparagraph (a) to provide an option in favour of the Purchaser to renew the said lease for two (2) further terms of five (5) years each in duration, provided that the Purchaser shall give the Lessor at least six (6) months' written notice of the desire to exercise such option on the same terms and conditions as contained in the said lease, save and except for the basic rent payable thereunder which shall be agreed upon between the Lessor and the Purchaser acting reasonably and having regard to the market rents for similar premises in the City of Anyville not less than three (3) months prior to the expiry of the then existing term; failing which the lease shall terminate on the then termination date.

(c) Notwithstanding the generality of the foregoing, it shall be a condition of this Offer that the Vendor obtain the written consent of the Lessor to amend the terms of the existing lease referred to in subparagraph (a) to provide that, upon the Purchaser vacating the premises for any reason, the Lessor agrees that he shall not, for a period of two (2) years, lease the premises vacated by the Purchaser for the purposes of the carrying on of a veterinary practice, and that during the term of the lease or any renewal term the Purchaser shall have the exclusive right to carry on a veterinary practice in the building or buildings of which the leased premises form a part.

8.00   Vendor's Warranties and Covenants

8.01   The Vendor represents and warrants that she is the owner of the Practice and assets herein agreed to be purchased, and that the same are free and clear of all liens and encumbrances whatsoever, except as aforesaid.

8.02   The Vendor represents and warrants that all statements contained in this Offer are true in fact and substance and that the financial statements shown to the Purchaser are correct and accurate and have been prepared in accordance with generally accepted accounting principles applied on a consistent basis.

8.03   The Vendor covenants and agrees to advise Bell Canada that she does not require the telephone number allocated for the Practice purchased herein and consents to the continued use of that number by the Purchaser.

8.04   The Vendor agrees to comply with Section 4 of The Retail Sales Tax Act.

8.05   The Vendor warrants, which warranty shall survive the completion of this transaction, that she is a registrant pursuant to the provisions of the Excise Tax Act (Canada) and that the transaction contemplated herein constitutes a taxable supply of substantially all of the assets of the business for which Goods and Services Tax ("G.S.T.") will be exigible and agrees to execute a form of election pursuant to Section 167 of the Excise Tax Act electing to exempt the within transaction from the payment of G.S.T.

8.06   The Vendor agrees to employ the Purchaser as an employee veterinarian of the Practice for the period commencing the 2nd day of July, 1994 and ending on the closing date herein at a salary based on FIFTY THOUSAND ($50,000.00) dollars per annum. The Purchaser shall be required to perform all of the usual duties and functions of a veterinary practitioner during the term of this employment engagement.

8.07   The Vendor agrees to remain on the premises of the Practice for a period of two (2) months from the date of closing, without compensation, for the purpose of assisting the Purchaser in the transition of the Practice including, but not limited to, client introductions, review of patient files and accounting records and familiarity with practice equipment.

8.08   The Vendor will provide on closing a Statutory Declaration confirming the covenants, representations and warranties set out in this Agreement.

8.09   Notwithstanding the completion of this transaction, the covenants, representations and warranties on the part of the Vendor contained in this Agreement shall continue in full force and effect for the benefit of the Purchaser.

9.00   Vendor's Indemnity

9.01   The Vendor agrees to indemnify and save harmless the Purchaser from and against all accounts payable, liabilities, claims and demands whatsoever, including liabilities, claims and demands for income taxes, sales, excise or other taxes of or in connection with the said business, existing or accrued as at the effective date hereinbefore referred to.

9.02   The Vendor agrees to indemnify the Purchaser in respect of any monies paid or costs or damages incurred by the Purchaser for breach by the Vendor of any warranty, either expressed or implied, given by the Vendor to the Purchaser prior to or on the date of closing herein.

9.03   The Vendor agrees to enter into an agreement with the Purchaser in a form satisfactory to the solicitor for the Purchaser providing for such indemnities aforesaid.

10.00   Insurance

10.01   Until the date of closing, all buildings, equipment and inventory as herein defined shall be and remain at the risk of the Vendor and the Vendor shall hold all policies of insurance effected on the said property and assets and the proceeds of such insurance in trust for the parties hereto, as their interests may appear. In the event of damage to the building, equipment or inventory before the completion of this transaction, the Purchaser shall have the right to elect to take such proceeds and complete the purchase or cancel this Agreement. If the Agreement is cancelled, the Purchaser shall be entitled to the return, without interest, of all monies theretofore paid on account of this purchase. The Vendor shall provide the Purchaser with particulars of all policies of insurance on the business and premises for which the Vendor wishes to transfer to the Purchaser on closing at least five (5) days prior to closing. The Purchaser may elect to accept such transfers, or to place his own insurance, in which case there shall be no adjustment for insurance premiums.

11.00   Employees

11.01   The Purchaser hereby agrees to assume the employment of all of the employees and associates of the Practice on the same terms and conditions thereof as set out in Schedule "B" annexed to this Agreement.

12.00 Restriction on Competition

12.01 The Vendor covenants and agrees with the Purchaser, in consideration of the Purchaser purchasing the assets purchased hereunder from the Vendor, that the Vendor will execute and deliver to the Purchaser on the date of closing an agreement under seal that the Vendor shall not either alone or in association with any person, firm or corporation, and whether as principal, agent, shareholder or otherwise, directly or indirectly, be engaged in, carry on or be otherwise connected with or financially interested in any veterinary practice within the present limits of the City of Anyville and the radius thereof set out below for a period of five (5) years from the date of closing during the periods set opposite such radius:

Radius		Years from Closing
10	kilometres	1
8	kilometres	2
6	kilometres	3
4	kilometres	4
2	kilometres	5

13.00 General

13.01 This sale to be made under and subject to the provisions of The Bulk Sales Act.

13.02 The Purchaser shall be credited towards the purchase price with the amount, if any, which it shall be necessary for the Purchaser to pay to the Minister of National Revenue in order to satisfy the Purchaser's liability in respect of tax payable by the Vendor under the non-residency provisions of The Income Tax Act by reason of this sale. The Purchaser shall not claim such credit if the Vendor delivers on the date of closing the prescribed Certificate or her Statutory Declaration that she is not then a non-resident of Canada.

13.03   This Offer when accepted shall constitute a binding contract of purchase and sale, and time in all respects shall be of the essence of this Agreement.

13.04   The parties hereto agree that there is no representation, warranty, collateral agreement or condition affecting this Agreement or stipulated hereby other than as expressed herein in writing.

13.05   Any tender of documents or money hereunder may be made upon the Vendor or Purchaser or upon the solicitor acting for the party on whom tender is desired, and it shall be sufficient that a negotiable certified cheque is tendered instead of cash.

13.06   In the event of failure on the part of the Purchaser to carry out the terms hereof, the deposit is to be retained by the Vendor as liquidated damages and not as a penalty.

13.07   Section headings are not to be considered part of this Agreement and are included solely for convenience of reference and are not intended to be full or accurate descriptions of the contents thereof.

13.08   This Offer and its acceptance to be read with all changes of gender or number required by the context.

13.09   This Agreement shall enure to the benefit of and be binding upon the heirs, executors and administrators of the parties hereto. This Agreement shall not be assignable by either of the parties hereto without the prior written consent of the other party. All covenants on the part of more than one party shall be both joint and several.

13.10   All dollar amounts referred to in this Agreement are Canadian funds, unless otherwise provided.

13.11   The Vendor shall deliver such other documents as provided for in this Agreement or which may by notice in writing given to the Vendor or her solicitors prior to the date of closing be reasonably required by the Purchaser or his solicitors.

13.12   This Offer shall be irrevocable by the Purchaser until 5:00 p.m. on the 19th day of June, 1994, after which time, if not accepted, this Offer shall be null and void and the deposit returned to the Purchaser without interest or deduction.

DATED at Anywhere, this 17th day of June, 1994.

IN WITNESS WHEREOF the Purchaser has executed this Offer under seal.

SIGNED, SEALED
AND DELIVERED
in the presence of

_____

John White

_____
Witness

The undersigned Vendor hereby accepts the foregoing Offer.

DATED at Anyville, this 18th day of June, 1994.

IN WITNESS WHEREOF the Vendor has executed this Offer under seal.

SIGNED, SEALED
AND DELIVERED
in the presence of

_____

Jane Black

_____
Witness

SCHEDULE "A" to Agreement of Purchase and Sale between John White, as Purchaser, and Jane Black, as Vendor, Accepted by the Vendor on the 18th day of June, 1994.

List of Equipment and Chattels

[to be completed by the parties prior to closing]

SCHEDULE "B" to Agreement of Purchase and Sale between John White, as Purchaser, and Jane Black, as Vendor, accepted by the Vendor on the 18th day of June, 1994.

Employees and Their Terms of Employment

Employee Name	Date of Commencement of Employment	Hourly Wage	Benefits
Mary Brown	June 14, 1991	$15.00	Medical, Dental
Joseph Green	December 1, 1990	$15.00	None

APPENDIX C

Partnership Agreement

THIS AGREEMENT made the 5th day of February, 1994.

BETWEEN:

JOHN WHITE
(hereinafter referred to as "White")

OF THE FIRST PART

- and -

JANE BLACK
(hereinafter referred to as "Black")

OF THE SECOND PART

WHEREAS:

1.   White and Black wish to constitute themselves as partners for the purpose of carrying on a professional practice of veterinary medicine in accordance with the terms of these Articles;

2.   White and Black are the owners of certain items of machinery and equipment as set out in Schedule "A" annexed hereto each as to an undivided one-half partnership interest (the "Partnership Property");

3.   White and Black hold the degrees of Doctor of Veterinary Medicine and are members in good standing of the College of Veterinarians of Ontario;

4.   White and Black believe it to be in their mutual best interest to provide for continuity of ownership and control of the Partnership and to provide for certain rules respecting the conduct of the affairs of the Partnership and of the Partners with respect thereto.

NOW THEREFORE THIS AGREEMENT WITNESSETH that in consideration of the covenants, agreements and promises herein set forth and other good and valuable consideration, the receipt and sufficiency of which is by all the parties hereto acknowledged, THE PARTIES AGREE AS FOLLOWS:

1.00   CONSTITUTION OF PARTNERSHIP

1.01   Definitions

In these Articles the following definitions apply:

(a) "Partnership" shall be the Partnership constituted by these Articles;

(b) "Partnership Interest" shall be the share of a Partner in the Partnership as defined in Article 2.00;

(c) "Partner" shall mean either of White or Black.

1.02   Constitution

White and Black hereby constitute themselves a Partnership for the purpose of carrying on business from the 10th day of February, 1994, and the Partnership shall continue until determined in accordance with the Articles.

1.03   Name

(a) The name of the Partnership shall be "Fantasy Veterinary Services" or such other name as the Partners may agree upon.

(b) The name shall be property of the Partnership and neither Partner shall be entitled to use such name unless he or she shall remain a Partner of the Partnership, and in the event of dissolution of the Partnership, neither Partner shall use the name without the consent in writing of the other.

1.04   The Partnership Property shall be held in the names of the Partners as partnership property and shall be disposed of only in accordance with the terms of these Articles.

2.00   PROPORTIONATE INTEREST

2.01   Equal Shares

The Partners shall share in the assets of the Partnership in equal proportions, which shares are referred to herein as Partnership Interests. For greater certainty, each Partner shall have a fifty per cent (50%) interest in the Partnership.

3.00   MANAGEMENT

3.01   Partner Decisions

All Partnership decisions, not delegated by either of the Partners, shall be made by the majority of the Partners present at any meeting of the Partners, of which meeting notice has been given and which a quorum is present.

3.02   Partnership Meetings

The Partners shall meet on a monthly basis on the third (3rd) Tuesday of each month during the term of this Agreement, or at any other time upon request by either Partner.

3.03   Banking

The Partnership shall maintain bank accounts at the Royal Bank of Canada, or such other bank or financial institution as the Partners may, from time to time, agree and all funds received by the Partners shall be deposited into such accounts. Either Partner shall have the authority to sign cheques or other withdrawals from the Partnership accounts.

3.04   Attention

Each Partner agrees to devote his full time and attention to the affairs of the Partnership.

3.05   Accounting Records

The Partnership shall maintain adequate accounting records and all books, records and accounts of the Partnership shall at all times be open for inspection by either of the Partners.

3.06   Accountants

Until changed by the Partners, Number and Crunchers shall be appointed the Accountants of the Partnership.

3.07   Fiscal Year-End

The fiscal year-end of the Partnership shall be the 30th day of April in each year.

3.08   Partnership Draws

Each Partner shall receive such semi-monthly draw as shall be agreed upon from time to time by the Partners, with such draw to be credited against his or her Partnership Interest in the profits of the Partnership.

4.00   TRANSFER OR SALE OF INTEREST

4.01   Prohibition

Neither partner shall sell, assign, transfer, encumber, pledge or dispose of his or her interest in the Partnership without the written consent of the other Partner, except as herein provided.

4.02   New Partners

No further partners shall be admitted to the Partnership without the prior written consent of both Partners.

4.03   Profits and Losses

Profits and losses of the Partnership shall be allocated to the Partners in proportion to their respective Partnership Interest.

4.04   Sale of Partnership Property

In the event that the Partnership Property is disposed of, each Partner shall be entitled to receive from the net proceeds of any such sale a sum equal to his or her proportionate Partnership Interest.

4.05   Transfer to Outsiders — Right of First Negotiation

(a) **Offer to Sell** — If either of Black or White desires to transfer or sell all of his or her Partnership Interest in the Partnership, such Partner (in this Section called the "Offeror") shall first make an offer in writing to the other Partner (in this Section called the "Offeree") to sell his or her Partnership Interest to the Offeree. Such offer shall specify the total sale price, the manner of payment, the date of closing, and any other terms of sale, which offer shall be open for acceptance for a period of no less than thirty (30) days from delivery thereof (the "30-day period").

(b) **Deemed Terms** — If the offer is accepted by the Offeree, the Offeree may, by notice in writing given at the time of acceptance, deem that the agreement shall contain the following provisions:

   (i)   The purchase price shall be for cash without deferred payment or other consideration at the purchase price set forth;

   (ii)   The Partnership shall pay and discharge all indebtedness owing to the selling Partner in full on or before closing, and to the extent that the Partnership will be rendered insolvent by so doing, such indebtedness shall be purchased in full by the Purchaser;

   (iii) The Purchaser shall cause any guarantees given, liabilities assumed, or obligations incurred on behalf of the Partnership by the selling Partner to be delivered up and cancelled. If, in order to obtain such cancellations, the Purchaser or the Partnership shall be required to give any additional or further security or guarantees to the holder thereof, or to refinance any loans or indebtedness, it shall do so. If a cancellation is not available despite the Purchaser's best efforts, the Purchaser shall indemnify the selling Partner against and save him or her harmless from all claims arising out of such guarantees or other obligations.

(c) **Six-Month Period** — If the offer is not accepted by the Offeree, the Offeror may, within the six (6) months (the "6-month period") following expiry of the 30-day period, sell his or her Partnership Interest to any third party at a price not less than the price at which, and on terms not more favourable than, the terms on which such Partnership Interest was offered to the Offeree. If, within the 6-month period, the Offeror is prepared to accept an offer on terms less than the price at which, or more favourable than, the terms on which such Partnership Interest was offered by the Offeror, he or she may not accept such offer without delivering a true copy of the third party offer and a statement that the Offeror intends to accept such offer to the Offeree and without first re-offering the Partnership Interest on the same terms to the Offeree as set forth in Section 4.05(a) except that the 30-day period shall be reduced to fifteen (15) days.

(d) **Conditions Precedent to Transfer** — No transfer shall be permitted or recorded to a third party purchaser unless the following conditions are first fulfilled:

(i)   The provisions of this Section are complied with;

(ii)   a true copy of the accepted third-party offer between the Offeror and the third-party purchaser and a statutory declaration of the Offeror and the third-party purchaser that the transaction was completed in accordance with the terms of the accepted third-party offer is delivered to the Offeree;

(iii)   the third-party purchaser delivers to the Partnership a covenant under seal to be bound by and succeed to the rights and obligations of the Offeror under this Agreement except any rights related to personal service or employment of the Offeror.

(e) **Audit** — The Offeree shall have the right, at his or her own expense, to conduct an audit of the Partnership's books during the 30-day period, and all information received will be deemed to be confidential.

5.00   INCAPACITY OF A PARTNER

5.01   Effective on Incapacity

If either Partner should become incapacitated, the provisions of this Section shall apply.

5.02   Definition of Incapacity

Incapacity of a Partner shall be defined as incapacity due to accident or illness, be the same physical or mental illness, or other cause, resulting in the failure to attend to the business of the Partnership to the extent attended to by the said Partner prior to such incapacity, for a period of six (6) months out of nine (9) consecutive months, or resulting in an immediate, continuous and permanent mental or physical incapacity such that the Partner will be permanently unable to so attend to the business of the Partnership. A finding of mental incompetency or inability to manage one's affairs under The Mental Incompetency Act or similar statute shall be conclusive evidence of incompetency. The remaining Partner, if only one, shall, in writing within three (3) months after the Partner becomes incapacitated, fix a date within the three (3) months which shall be deemed the effective date of incapacity.

5.03   Resignations

An incapacitated Partner shall be deemed to have resigned as a partner at the time he or she is determined to be incapacitated.

5.04   Value of Investment

The value of the investment of the incapacitated Partner shall be determined by the Accountants of the Partnership who shall be at liberty to engage an independent business valuator. The determination of such value shall be binding upon all of the Partners.

5.05   Terms of Payment

(a) The payments by the Partnership and the remaining Partner shall be by cash or certified cheque in full on closing.

(b) Notwithstanding clause (a) above, the remaining Partner may at his or her option pay one-third (1/3) of the purchase price on such date and the balance by way of a promissory note in equal semi-annual instalments over a period of two (2) years with interest charged at the rate adjusted on the first day of each month to the prime commercial lending rate in effect at the Partnership's primary lending bank on such date plus two per cent (2%) per annum calculated, compounded and payable monthly.

5.06   Execution of Documents

Any receipts, releases and documents necessary to give effect to this Article shall be endorsed and signed by the guardian or committee, as the case may be, if any, of the incapacitated Partner, or if none then by his or her spouse, and if none then by the remaining Partner of the Partnership, it being agreed by all parties that such persons are hereby granted and given irrevocable authority to endorse and sign such receipts, releases and documents.

5.07   Closing

The transaction shall be closed on the thirtieth (30th) day following final determination of the value of the investment, or the last preceding banking day if such day is not a banking day.

6.00   TERMS OF SALE

6.01   The provisions of this Article apply to any sale or transfer of a Partnership Interest pursuant to Article 4.00 and Article 5.00 hereof; provided that the specific provisions of Article 4.00 and Article 5.00 shall prevail over the provisions hereof in the event of a conflict.

6.02 The closing of the transaction shall take place at the office of the solicitors for the Partnership at 2:00 o'clock in the afternoon on the date fixed for closing.

6.03 On closing, the selling Partner shall deliver the following:

(a) the resignation of the selling Partner or his/her nominee as a Partner of the Partnership;

(b) a release to the Partnership and the purchaser of any and all claims he or she may have against the Partnership and the purchaser in respect of loss of office as officer or out of any employment agreement which he or she may have entered into with the Partnership other than with respect to accrued salaries and benefits;

(c) a release to the purchaser and the Partnership from the provisions of this Agreement save as to those provisions specifically stated to continue after termination of this Agreement;

(d) promissory notes and other evidences of indebtedness acquired by the purchaser, duly endorsed and transferred, together with all security held in connection therewith;

(e) an undertaking to give such further assurances and do all other things required in order to deliver title to the Partnership Interest and indebtedness acquired by the purchaser free and clear of claims of all others;

(f) such additional undertakings, covenants, warranties and guarantees that are provided by this Agreement to survive termination of the Agreement;

(g) a covenant that the selling Partner is the owner with good and marketable title, free of any encumbrances and liens of any kind, of the Partnership Interest, indebtedness, loans and other property acquired by the purchaser, and that the selling Partner has the exclusive right and full power to sell, transfer and assign the said property to the purchaser; and,

(h) a covenant from the selling Partner that he or she will not, either alone or as an employee, partner or in any other manner, practise veterinary medicine or surgery for a period of two (2) years in the City of Anywhere, or within a radius of one hundred (100) kilometres thereof.

6.04 On closing, the purchaser will deliver to the selling Partner the following:

(a) the balance of funds due on closing;

(b) an indemnity with respect to any personal guarantees given by the selling Partner on behalf of the Partnership;

(c) a release from this Agreement except those provisions hereof as are provided will survive the termination of the Agreement; and,

(d) such other assurances, documents and instruments as the selling Partner or his/her solicitor may reasonably require to give effect to the foregoing and the intent of this Agreement.

6.05 The Partnership and the purchaser shall have the right to set off against any sums of money due to the selling Partner of the amount of any indebtedness of the Partner to the Partnership or the purchaser, notwithstanding that such indebtedness shall not then have matured and be due and payable. Furthermore, the purchaser shall be entitled to pay the Partnership the amount of any indebtedness of the selling Partner to the Partnership and the Partnership shall be entitled to pay the purchaser the amount of any indebtedness of the selling Partner to the purchaser, and the amount of such payment may be set off against any amounts due to the selling Partner by the Partnership or the purchaser.

6.06 The selling Partner hereby irrevocably appoints the purchaser his/her lawful attorney for purposes of this section. The purchaser hereby irrevocably appoints the selling Partner his/her lawful attorney for purposes of this section. If either the purchaser or the selling Partner shall neglect or refuse to attend at closing and deliver the transfers, instruments and other documents provided herein, the attorney is authorized to execute and deliver all such transfers, instruments and documents on behalf of and in the name of his/her principal and the principal hereby ratifies and confirms all such acts by his/her attorney; provided that the attorney forthwith delivers to his/her principal true copies of all such transfers, instruments and documents as executed.

6.07 Any tender of monies shall be sufficient if made by certified cheque or bank draft drawn on a Canadian chartered bank, and any tender may be made upon the parties or their respective solicitors.

7.00   DISSOLUTION

7.01   Notice

(a) The Partnership may be dissolved upon three (3) months' notice in writing by either Partner to the other.

(b) Upon dissolution, the Partnership Property and all other assets of the Partnership shall be disposed of in an orderly fashion as may be agreed upon by the Partners. Either Partner shall be entitled to purchase any of the assets of the Partnership upon dissolution.

8.00   GENERAL

8.01   Termination of Agreement

This Agreement shall terminate upon the occurrence of any one of the following events:

(a) voluntary agreement in writing of the Partners;

(b) cessation of the Partnership's business and distribution of all the Partnership's assets between the Partners;

(c) with respect to either Partner, upon the sale or transfer by him/her of all his/her Partnership Interest in the Partnership; and,

(d) with respect to either Partner, upon his/her ceasing to be a member in good standing of the College of Veterinarians of Ontario, or immediately upon a finding by any discipline committee of the College of Veterinarians of Ontario of conduct unbecoming of a member of such Association.

8.02   Notice

Any Notice authorized or required by this Agreement to be given or served shall be in writing and deemed to be duly given or served if the same shall be delivered personally, or shall be sent by prepaid registered mail with return receipt requested addressed to a Partner at the addresses set out below, and if so sent shall be conclusively deemed to have been given on the third (3rd) business day after the date of mailing:

In the case of White at:

900 Imagine Avenue
Anywhere, Ontario   N1H 2Z4

In the case of Black at:

326 Nowhere Crescent
Anywhere, Ontario   N1H 3P1

8.03 **Amendment to Agreement**

This Agreement may be altered or amended at any time by the written agreement of all of the parties hereto.

8.04 **Assignment**

The interest of either Partner under this Agreement shall not be assigned to any person without the consent in writing of the other Partner hereto.

8.05 **Waiver**

A waiver by either Partner of any of his/her rights or of the performance of the other Partner of any of his/her obligations under this Agreement shall be without prejudice to all or any of his/her other rights under the Agreement.

8.06 **Governing Law**

This Agreement shall be governed by and construed in accordance with the laws of the Province of Ontario.

8.07 **Entire Agreement**

This Agreement constitutes the entire agreement between the Partners and there are no representations or warranties or other terms except as herein contained in writing.

8.08 **Counterparts**

This Agreement may be executed in several counterparts each of which so executed shall be deemed to be an original and such counterparts together shall constitute one and the same instrument.

8.09 **Time of the Essence**

Time shall in all respects be of the essence of this Agreement.

8.10 **Enurement**

This Agreement shall enure to the benefit of and be binding upon the parties hereto and their respective heirs, executors, administrators and assigns.

IN WITNESS WHEREOF the parties have duly executed this Agreement under seal.

SIGNED, SEALED
AND DELIVERED
in the presence of

_____	_____
Witness	**John White**
_____	_____
Witness	**Jane Black**

APPENDIX D

Provincial Statutes

Province	Statute
Alberta	Veterinary Profession Act
British Columbia	Veterinarians Act
Manitoba	Veterinary Medical Act
New Brunswick	Veterinarians Act
Newfoundland and Labrador	Veterinary Medical Act
Northwest Territories	Veterinary Profession Act
Nova Scotia	Veterinary Medical Act
Ontario	Veterinarians Act
Prince Edward Island	Veterinary Profession Act
Quebec	Professional Code Veterinary Surgeons Act
Saskatchewan	Veterinarians Act

APPENDIX E

Governing Bodies

Alberta Veterinary Medical Association
Suite 100,
8615 — 149th Street,
Edmonton, Alberta
T5R 1B3

British Columbia Veterinary Medical Association
Suite 155,
1200 West 73rd Street,
Vancouver, British Columbia
V6P 6G5

Veterinary Medical Board of Manitoba
Veterinary Services Branch,
545 University Crescent,
Winnipeg, Manitoba
R3T 5S6

Corporation Professionelle des Médecins Vétérinaires du Québec
795 Avenue du Palais,
Suite 200,
St. Hyacinthe, Québec
J2S 5C6

Saskatchewan Veterinary Medical Association
Suite 104,
112 Research Drive,
Saskatoon, Saskatchewan
S7N 3R3

New Brunswick Veterinary Medical Association,
P.O. Box 1065,
Moncton, New Brunswick
E1C 8P2

Nova Scotia Veterinary Medical Association
15 Cobequid Road,
Lower Sackville, Nova Scotia
B4C 2M9

College of Veterinarians of Ontario
R. R. # 3,
Guelph, Ontario
N1H 6H9

Prince Edward Island Veterinary Medical Association
Agriculture Canada
P.O. Box 100,
Montague, Prince Edward Island
C0A 1R0

Newfoundland and Labrador Veterinary Licensing Board,
Ministry of Agriculture and Food,
P.O. Box 569,
Harbour Grace, Newfoundland
A0A 2M0

APPENDIX F

Veterinarians Act (Ontario), RSO 1990, c. V.3

CONTENTS

Definitions

1.—(1) In this Act,

"Board" means the Health Disciplines Board under the *Health Disciplines Act*; ("Conseil")

"by-laws" means the by-laws made under this Act; ("règlements administratifs")

"certificate of accreditation" means a certificate of accreditation issued under this Act to establish or operate a veterinary facility; ("certificat d'agrément")

"College" means the College of Veterinarians of Ontario; ("Ordre")

"Council" means the Council of the College; ("conseil")

"drug" means drug as defined in Part VI of the *Health Disciplines Act*; ("médicament")

"impaired", in relation to a person, means suffering from a physical or mental condition or disorder of a nature and extent that adversely affects the person's ability to practice veterinary medicine; ("affaibli")

"licence" means a licence to engage in the practice of veterinary medicine issued under this Act; ("permis")

"Minister" means the Minister of Agriculture and Food; ("ministre")

"practice of veterinary medicine" includes the practice of dentistry, obstetrics including ova and embryo transfer, and surgery, in relation to an animal other than a human being; ("exercice de la médecine vétérinaire")

"Registrar" means the Registrar of the College; ("registrateur")

"regulations" means the regulations made under this Act; ("règlements")

"veterinary facility" means a building, land or vehicle or any combination of them used or intended to be used as a place in or from which to engage in the practice of veterinary medicine. ("établissement vétérinaire")

Hearings and submissions

(2) Despite the *Statutory Powers Procedure Act*, no board, committee, person or group of persons shall be required to hold a hearing or to afford to any person an opportunity to appear or to make submissions before making a decision or proposal, giving a direction or otherwise disposing of a matter under this Act except to the extent that a hearing or an opportunity to appear or to make submissions is specifically required by this Act. 1989, c. 60, s. 1.

Name

2. The Ontario Veterinary Association, a body corporate, is continued as a corporation without share capital under the name College of Veterinarians of Ontario in English and the name Ordre des vétérinaires de l'Ontario in French. 1989, c. 60, s. 2, *revised*.

Objects

3.—(1) The principal object of the College is to regulate the practice of veterinary medicine and to govern its members in accordance with this Act, the regulations and the by-laws in order that the public interest may be served and protected.

Idem

(2) For the purpose of carrying out its principal object, the College has the following additional objects:

1. To establish, maintain and develop standards of knowledge and skill among its members.

2. To establish, maintain and develop standards of qualification and standards of practice for the practice of veterinary medicine.

3. To establish, maintain and develop standards of professional ethics among its members.

4. To promote public awareness of the role of the College.

5. To perform such other duties and exercise such other powers as are imposed or conferred on the College under any Act.

Capacity and powers of College

(3) For the purpose of carrying out its objects, the College has the capacity and the powers of a natural person. 1989, c. 60, s. 3.

Council

4.—(1) The council of the Ontario Veterinary Association is continued as the Council of the College and shall be the governing body and board of directors of the College and shall manage and administer its affairs.

Composition

(2) The Council shall be composed of,

(a) not fewer than nine and not more than fifteen persons who are members of the College and are elected by the members of the College in the number and manner provided by by-law of the Council; and

(b) not fewer than three and not more than five persons who are not members of the governing body of a self-regulating licensing body under any other Act or licensed under this Act and who are appointed by the Lieutenant Governor in Council.

Remuneration of lay members

(3) The persons appointed under clause (2) (b) shall be paid, out of the money appropriated therefor by the Legislature, such expenses and remuneration as are determined by the Lieutenant Governor in Council.

Term of office

(4) The term of an appointment under clause (2) (b) must not exceed three years.

Reappointment

(5) A person whose appointment under clause (2) (b) expires is eligible for reappointment but no person shall be appointed and reappointed for more than six consecutive years.

Qualifications

(6) Every member of the College who,

(a) practises or resides in Ontario;

(b) is the holder of a licence that is not limited to the practice of veterinary medicine for educational purposes only;

(c) is not in default of an annual fee prescribed by the regulations; and

(d) is not in default of filing a return required by the regulations, is qualified to vote at an election of members of the Council for the constituency to which the member of the College belongs.

Officers

(7) The Council shall elect annually a president and one or more vice-presidents of the College from among the elected members of the Council.

Registrar and staff

(8) The Council shall appoint a Registrar, and the Executive Committee may appoint such other persons as are from time to time necessary or desirable in the opinion of the Executive Committee to perform the work of the College.

Quorum

(9) A majority of the members of the Council constitutes a quorum.

Vacancies

(10) Where one or more vacancies occur in the membership of the Council, the members remaining in office constitute the Council so long as their number is not fewer than a quorum.

Continuation of council members

(11) The members of the council of the Ontario Veterinary Association who were in office immediately before the 4th day of April, 1990 shall continue in office until the expiration of their terms or until their offices otherwise become vacant. 1989, c. 60, s. 4.

Membership

5.—(1) Every person who holds a licence is a member of the College subject to any conditions and limitations to which the licence is subject.

Resignation of membership

(2) A member may resign his or her membership by filing with the Registrar a resignation in writing and the member's licence is thereupon cancelled.

Cancellation for default of fees

(3) The Registrar may cancel a licence for non-payment of any fee prescribed by the regulations or for failure to file a return required by the regulations after giving the member at least two months notice of the default and intention to cancel.

Continuing jurisdiction

(4) A person whose licence is cancelled, revoked or suspended remains subject to the continuing jurisdiction of the College in respect of,

(a) an investigation or disciplinary action arising out of his or her conduct while a member; and

(b) an inquiry or proceeding related to whether the person is impaired. 1989, c. 60, s. 5.

Powers of Minister

6. In addition to the Minister's other powers and duties under this Act, the Minister may,

(a) review the activities of the Council;

(b) request the Council to undertake activities that, in the opinion of the Minister, are necessary and advisable to carry out the intent of this Act;

(c) advise the Council with respect to the implementation of this Act and the regulations and with respect to the methods used or proposed to be used by the Council to implement policies and to enforce its regulations and procedures;

(d) request the Council to make, amend or revoke regulations respecting any matter under section 7 or the standards for veterinary facilities established under section 8. 1989, c. 60, s. 6.

Regulations

7.—(1) Subject to the approval of the Lieutenant Governor in Council and with prior review by the Minister, the Council may make regulations with respect to the following matters:

1. Prescribing classes of licences and governing the qualifications and requirements for the issuance of licences or any class thereof and prescribing the conditions and limitations thereof.

2. Respecting any matter ancillary to the provisions of this Act with regard to the issuance, cancellation, suspension and revocation of licences.

3. Respecting any matter ancillary to the provisions of this Act with regard to the issuance, renewal, suspension and revocation of certificates of accreditation.

4. Prescribing classes of certificates of accreditation and governing the qualifications and requirements for the issuance and renewal of certificates of accreditation or any class thereof and prescribing the conditions and limitations thereof.

5. Providing for the designation of members of the College as specialists, prescribing the qualifications and requirements for designation as a specialist, providing for the suspension or revocation of such a designation and for the regulation and prohibition of the use of the designation by members of the College.

6. Governing the use of names and designations in the practice of veterinary medicine by members of the College.

7. Authorizing entries in, and the form of maintenance of, registers of members and former members of the College and directories of veterinary facilities and providing for the issuance of certificates of standing by the Registrar.

8. Prescribing and governing standards of practice for the profession.

9. Regulating the compounding, dispensing and sale of drugs by members of the College, and the containers and labelling of drugs compounded, dispensed or sold by members, and prescribing the records that shall be kept in respect of such compounding, dispensing and sale.

10. Establishing a special category of membership for retired members and determining the rights, privileges, duties and obligations of such members.

11. Respecting the promotion or advertising of the practice of veterinary medicine.

12. Prohibiting the practice of veterinary medicine where there is a conflict of interest and defining conflict of interest for the purpose.

13. Defining professional misconduct for the purposes of this Act.

14. Respecting the reporting and publication of decisions in disciplinary matters.

15. Requiring the payment of annual fees by members of the College, fees for processing applications, licensing, certificates, examinations and inspections, including penalties for late payment, prompt payment discounts and interest on late payments and fees for anything the Registrar is required or authorized to do, and prescribing the amounts thereof.

16. Requiring the making of returns of information by members of the College in respect of names, addresses, telephone numbers, professional associates, partners, employees and professional activities.

17. Providing for the compilation of statistical information on the supply, distribution, professional liability insurance and professional activities of members of the College and requiring members to provide the information necessary to compile such statistics.

18. Requiring and providing for the inspection of veterinary facilities and of the records kept by members of the College in connection with the practice of veterinary medicine.

19. Authorizing the communication of material that comes to a person's knowledge in the course of duties, employment, examination, review or investigation to specified classes of persons or for specified purposes.

20. Respecting the duties and authority of the Registrar.

21. Prescribing and requiring the making and keeping of records by members of the College in respect of the practice of veterinary medicine.

22. Exempting any member of the College from any provision of the regulations under such special circumstances in the public interest as the Council considers advisable.

23. Providing that any form required under this Act be in a form approved by the Registrar.

Application (2) A regulation made under subsection (1) may be general or particular in its application.

Adoption of accreditation (3) For the purpose of prescribing the qualifications and requirements for the issuance of licences or the issuance and renewal of certificates of accreditation, the Council, in a regulation under subsection (1) or a standard under subsection 8 (1), may adopt as its own the recognition or accreditation granted by any organization specified by the Council.

Distribution of regulations (4) The Council shall,

(a) forward a copy of each regulation made under subsection (1) to each member of the College; and

(b) keep a copy of each regulation made under subsection (1) available for public inspection in the office of the College.

Regulations by Lieutenant Governor in Council (5) Where the Minister requests in writing under clause 6 (d) that the Council make, amend or revoke a regulation or standard and the Council has failed to do so within sixty days after the request, the Lieutenant Governor in Council may make regulations respecting the subject-matter set out in the request.

Conflicting provisions (6) In cases of conflict, a regulation made under subsection (5) prevails over a regulation or standard made under subsection (1) or 8 (1) respectively. 1989, c. 60, s. 7.

Standards for veterinary facilities **8.**—(1) The Council may establish standards for veterinary facilities not inconsistent with this Act and the regulations which must be met in order to qualify for the issuance or renewal of a certificate of accreditation or any class thereof.

Distribution of standards (2) The Council shall forward a copy of the standards established under subsection (1) to the Minister and to each member of the College and shall keep a copy available for public inspection in the office of the College. 1989, c. 60, s. 8.

By-laws **9.**—(1) The Council may pass by-laws relating to the administrative and domestic affairs of the College not inconsistent with this Act and the regulations and, without limiting the generality of the foregoing, may pass by-laws respecting the following matters:

1. Prescribing the seal and other insignia of the College and providing for their use.

2. Providing for the execution of documents by the College.

3. Respecting banking and finance.

4. Fixing the financial year of the College and providing for the audit of the accounts and transactions of the College.

5. Prescribing the number of vice-presidents of the College, prescribing procedures for the election of the president and vice-presidents and for the filling of vacancies in those offices.

6. Respecting the calling, holding and conducting of meetings of the Council and the duties of members of the Council.

7. Respecting the calling, holding and conducting of meetings of the membership of the College.

8. Providing for the remuneration of members of the Council and members of committees other than members appointed by the Lieutenant Governor in Council, and providing for payment of necessary expenses of the Council and committees in the conduct of their business.

9. Providing for the appointment, composition, powers, duties and quorums of additional or special committees.

10. Providing for the appointment of persons to make investigations for the purposes of this Act.

11. Providing procedures for the making, amending and revoking of by-laws.

12. Respecting management of the property of the College.

13. Respecting the application of the funds of the College and the investment and reinvestment of any of its funds not immediately required, and for the safekeeping of its securities.

14. Respecting the borrowing of money by the College and the giving of security therefor.

15. Respecting membership of the College in other organizations the objects of which are not inconsistent with and are complementary to those of the College, the payment of annual assessments and provision for representatives at meetings.

16. Delegating to the Executive Committee the powers and duties set out in the by-laws, but this paragraph does not authorize the delegation of the power to make, amend or revoke a regulation or a by-law.

17. Fixing the number of members to be elected to the Council under clause 4 (2) (a) and defining constituencies, and prescribing the number of representatives.

18. Respecting and governing the qualifications, nomination, election and term or terms of office of the members to be elected to the Council, and controverted elections.

19. Prescribing the conditions disqualifying elected members from sitting on the Council and governing the filling of vacancies on the Council.

Signed by-laws and resolutions (2) A by-law or resolution of the Council signed by a majority of the members of the Council is as valid as if passed at a meeting of the Council held for that purpose.

Confirmation of by-laws (3) A by-law passed by the Council is not effective until confirmed by the members of the College at a meeting or by means of a vote conducted by mail.

Distribution of by-laws (4) The Council shall,

(a) forward a copy of each by-law confirmed under subsection (3) to the Minister and to each member of the College; and

(b) keep a copy of each by-law confirmed under subsection (3) available for public inspection in the office of the College. 1989, c. 60, s. 9 (1-4).

Establishment of committees **10.**—(1) The following committees are hereby established:

1. Executive Committee.

2. Accreditation Committee.

3. Registration Committee.

4. Complaints Committee.

5. Discipline Committee.

Idem (2) The Council shall appoint the committees referred to in subsection (1) and may establish and appoint such other committees as it considers necessary.

Vacancies (3) Where one or more vacancies occur in the membership of a committee, the members remaining in office constitute the committee so long as their number is not fewer than the prescribed quorum.

Person to chair (4) The Council shall name one member of each committee to chair the committee.

Term (5) No. person shall be appointed and reappointed to the same committee for more than six consecutive years. 1989, c. 60, s. 10.

Licence required **11.**—(1) No person shall engage in the practice of veterinary medicine or hold himself, herself or itself out as engaging in the practice of veterinary medicine unless the person is the holder of a licence.

Exceptions (2) Subsection (1) does not apply to prevent a person,

(a) from rendering first aid or temporary assistance in an emergency without fee;

(b) from treating an animal if the person is the owner of the animal, is a member of the household of the owner of the animal or is employed for general agricultural or domestic work by the owner of the animal;

(c) from taking blood samples;

(d) from preventing or treating fish and invertebrate diseases;

(e) from collecting or using semen under the authority of a licence issued under the *Artificial Insemination of Livestock Act*;

(f) from collecting or transporting ova and embryos of animals other than mammals.

Idem, student (3) Subsection (1) does not apply to a student of veterinary medicine to the extent that the student is engaging in the undergraduate curriculum of studies at the Ontario Veterinary College of the University of Guelph.

Interpretation of owner (4) For the purpose of clause (2) (b), a person is not the owner of an animal if the person buys the animal, treats it and resells it or intended to resell it to either the person who sold it to him or her or to that person's nominee.

Proof of practice (5) For the purposes of this section, proof of the performance of one act in the practice of veterinary medicine on one occasion is sufficient to establish engaging in the practice of veterinary medicine.

Application of Part VI of *Health Disciplines Act* (6) Part VI of the *Health Disciplines Act* does not apply to prevent a person who holds a licence from compounding, dispensing or selling drugs in the course of engaging in the practice of veterinary medicine.

Sale of drugs (7) The *Livestock Medicines Act* does not apply to prevent a person who holds a licence from selling a drug in the course of engaging in the practice of veterinary medicine to an owner of livestock for the treatment of livestock. 1989, c. 60, s. 11.

Executive Committee **12.**—(1) The Executive Committee shall be composed of five members of the Council, including,

(a) the president and one or two vice-presidents of the College; and

(b) not more than three other members of the Council of whom one shall be a member of the Council appointed to the Council by the Lieutenant Governor in Council.

Quorum

(2) Three members of the Executive Committee constitute a quorum.

Functions

(3) The Executive Committee shall perform such functions of the Council as are delegated to it by the Council, the by-laws or this Act.

Other functions

(4) Subject to ratification by the Council at its next meeting, the Executive Committee, between meetings of the Council, may perform any other function of the Council that, in the opinion of the Executive Committee, must be performed immediately.

Limitation

(5) Subsection (4) does not apply to authorize the Executive Committee to make, amend or revoke a regulation, a by-law or a standard described under subsection 8 (1). 1989, c. 60, s. 12.

Registration Committee

13.—(1) The Registration Committee shall be composed of five persons of whom,

(a) not fewer than three shall be members of the Council elected to the Council by the members of the College;

(b) one shall be a member of the Council appointed to the Council by the Lieutenant Governor in Council; and

(c) one may be a member of the College who is not a member of the Council.

Quorum

(2) Three members of the Registration Committee constitute a quorum. 1989, c. 60, s. 13.

Issuance of licence

14.—(1) Subject to subsections (2) and (3), the Registrar shall issue a licence to any person who applies therefor in accordance with the regulations and who meets the qualifications and requirements prescribed by the regulations.

Grounds for refusal

(2) The Registrar shall refuse to issue a licence where, in the opinion of the Registrar,

(a) the applicant does not meet the qualifications and requirements for the issuance of the licence;

(b) the past conduct of the applicant affords reasonable ground for believing that the applicant will not engage in the practice of veterinary medicine with honesty and integrity; or

(c) there is reasonable ground for believing that the applicant is impaired.

Referral to Registration Committee

(3) The Registrar, on his or her own initiative, may refer and on the request of the applicant shall refer the application to the Registration Committee for a determination as to any of the matters mentioned in clauses (2) (a), (b) and (c).

Power of Registration Committee

(4) The Registration Committee shall determine the eligibility of applicants for licences referred to the Registration Committee under subsection (3) and may in any case require an applicant to obtain such additional experience, education or training as the Registration Committee specifies.

Exemption

(5) The Registration Committee may exempt an applicant from compliance with any qualification or requirement for a licence.

Directions to Registrar

(6) The Registration Committee, after considering an application for a licence, may direct the Registrar,

(a) to issue the licence;

(b) to refuse to issue the licence; or

(c) to issue the licence subject to the conditions and limitations the Registration Committee specifies. 1989, c. 60, s. 14.

Certificate of accreditation required

15. No person shall establish or operate a veterinary facility except under and in accordance with a certificate of accreditation. 1989, c. 60, s. 15.

Accreditation Committee

16.—(1) The Accreditation Committee shall be composed of five persons of whom,

(a) not fewer than three shall be members of the Council elected to the Council by the members of the College;

(b) one shall be a member of the Council appointed to the Council by the Lieutenant Governor in Council; and

(c) one may be a member of the College who is not a member of the Council.

Quorum

(2) Three members of the Accreditation Committee constitute a quorum. 1989, c. 60, s. 16.

Issuance of certificate of accreditation

17.—(1) Subject to subsections (2) and (3), the Registrar shall issue or renew a certificate of accreditation upon the application of a member of the College who applies therefor if the applicant and the veterinary facility meet the qualifications, requirements and standards prescribed by the regulations and by the Council for the proposed veterinary facility.

Grounds for refusal

(2) The Registrar shall refuse to issue or renew a certificate of accreditation where, in the opinion of the Registrar, the applicant or the veterinary facility does not meet the qualifications, requirements and standards prescribed by the regulations and by the Council for the proposed veterinary facility.

Referral to Accreditation Committee

(3) The Registrar, on his or her own initiative, may refer and on the request of the applicant shall refer the application to the Accreditation Committee for a determination as to whether or not the applicant or the facility or both meet the qualifications, requirements and standards prescribed by the regulations and by the Council for the proposed veterinary facility.

Exemption

(4) The Accreditation Committee may exempt an applicant or veterinary facility from compliance with any qualification, requirement or standard for a certificate of accreditation.

Directions to Registrar

(5) The Accreditation Committee shall determine the eligibility of applicants and facilities for certificates of accreditation that are referred to the Accreditation Committee under subsection (3) and, after considering an application for the issuance or renewal of a certificate of accreditation, may direct the Registrar,

(a) to issue or to renew the certificate of accreditation;

(b) to refuse to issue or to renew the certificate of accreditation; or

(c) to issue or to renew the certificate of accreditation subject to the conditions and limitations the Accreditation Committee specifies. 1989, c. 60, s. 17.

Hearing by Board

18.—(1) Where,

(a) the Registration Committee proposes to direct the Registrar to refuse to issue a licence or proposes to direct the Registrar to issue a licence subject to conditions or limitations; or

(b) the Accreditation Committee proposes to direct the Registrar to refuse to issue or to refuse to renew a certificate of accreditation, or proposes to direct the Registrar to issue or to renew a certificate of accreditation subject to conditions or limitations,

the Registrar on behalf of the committee shall serve notice of the proposal, together with written reasons therefor, on the applicant and shall send a copy of the proposal and the written reasons to the Board.

Exception

(2) Subsection (1) does not apply in respect of a proposal to refuse to issue a licence where the applicant previously held a licence that was suspended or revoked as a result of a decision of the Discipline Committee, a decision of the Registration Committee or a decision of the council of the Ontario Veterinary Association under a predecessor of this Act.

Right to a hearing or review

(3) The applicant is entitled to a hearing by the Board, or to a review by the Board of his or her application and documentary evidence in support thereof without oral evidence, if the applicant mails or delivers within fifteen days after the notice under subsection (1) is served on the applicant, notice in writing to the Board requiring the hearing or the review by the Board, as the applicant specifies.

Notice of right to hearing or review

(4) The notice under subsection (1) shall inform the applicant of the right to a hearing or review by the Board as set out in subsection (3).

Powers of committee where no hearing or review

(5) Where an applicant does not require a hearing or review by the Board in accordance with subsection (3), the Board shall so notify the committee making the proposal and the committee may carry out the proposal stated in its notice under subsection (1).

Hearing by Board

(6) Where an applicant requires a hearing by the Board in accordance with subsection (3), the Board shall appoint a time for, give notice of and hold the hearing.

Review by Board

(7) Where an applicant requires a review by the Board in accordance with subsection (3), the Board shall review the application and documentary evidence in support thereof without oral evidence.

Findings of fact

(8) The findings of fact of the Board pursuant to a hearing or review shall be based exclusively on evidence admissible or matters that may be noticed under sections 15 and 16 of the *Statutory Powers Procedure Act*.

Quorum

(9) Three members of the Board constitute a quorum for the purpose of a proceeding under this section.

Powers of Board re licence

(10) The Board shall, after the hearing or review in respect of a licence,

(a) confirm the proposed decision of the Registration Committee;

(b) require the Registration Committee to direct the Registrar to issue a licence of the appropriate class subject to such conditions and limitations as the Board considers appropriate in cases where the Board finds that the applicant meets the qualifications and requirements for registration and that the Committee has exercised its powers improperly; or

(c) refer the matter back to the Registration Committee for further consideration, and the Board may make such recommendations as it considers appropriate in the circumstances.

Powers of Board re certificate of accreditation

(11) The Board shall, after the hearing or review in respect of a certificate of accreditation,

(a) confirm the proposed decision of the Accreditation Committee;

(b) require the Accreditation Committee to direct the Registrar to issue or renew a certificate of accreditation for the appropriate class of veterinary facility subject to such conditions and limitations as the Board considers appropriate in cases where the Board finds that the applicant and the veterinary facility meet the qualifications, requirements and standards for the issuance or renewal of the certificate of accreditation and that the Committee has exercised its powers improperly; or

(c) refer the matter back to the Accreditation Committee for further consideration, and the Board may make such recommendations as it considers appropriate in the circumstances.

Extension of time for requiring hearing

(12) The Board may extend the time for the giving of notice requiring a hearing by an applicant under this section before or after the expiration of such time where it is satisfied that there are apparent grounds for granting relief to the applicant and that there are reasonable grounds for applying for the extension, and the Board may give such directions as it considers proper consequent upon the extension.

Parties

(13) The College and the applicant who has required the hearing are parties to proceedings before the Board under this section.

Prohibitions on publication and identification

(14) Section 29, which relates to proceedings of the Discipline Committee, applies with necessary modifications to a hearing by the Board under this section.

Examination of documentary evidence

(15) A party to a hearing under this section shall be afforded an opportunity to examine before the hearing any written or documentary evidence that will be produced or any report the contents of which will be given in evidence at the hearing.

<table>
<tr><td>Members holding hearing or review not to have taken part in investigation, etc.</td><td>(16) Members of the Board holding a hearing or review shall not have taken part before the hearing or review in any investigation or consideration of the subject-matter of the hearing or review other than at a previous hearing or review of the Board and shall not communicate directly or indirectly in relation to the subject-matter of the hearing or review with any person or with any party or any party's representative except upon notice to and opportunity for all parties to participate, but the Board may seek legal advice from an adviser independent from the parties and, in such case, the nature of the advice shall be made known to the parties in order that they may make submissions as to the law. 1989, c. 60, s. 18 (1-16).</td></tr>
</table>

Recording of evidence

(17) The oral evidence taken before the Board at a hearing shall be recorded and, if so required, copies of a transcript of the oral evidence shall be furnished upon the same terms as in the Ontario Court (General Division). 1989, c. 60, s. 18 (17), *revised*.

Only members at hearing to participate in decision

(18) No member of the Board shall participate in a decision of the Board following upon a hearing unless he or she was present throughout the hearing and heard the evidence and argument of the parties.

Release of documentary evidence

(19) Documents and things put in evidence at a hearing shall, upon the request of the person who produced them, be released to the person within a reasonable time after the matter in issue has been finally determined. 1989, c. 60, s. 18 (18, 19).

Registers

19.—(1) The Registrar shall maintain one or more registers in which is entered,

(a) the name of every person to whom a licence is issued;

(b) any designation of a member of the College as a specialist and any withdrawal of recognition of the member's specialist status;

(c) any conditions or limitations imposed on a licence by a committee;

(d) any revocation, suspension, cancellation or termination of a licence;

(e) the fact and amount of a fine imposed by the Discipline Committee and the fact of a reprimand by the Discipline Committee, unless the Discipline Committee directs that no entry be made;

(f) where an entry results from a decision of a committee, the name of the committee that made the decision and any finding of the committee resulting in the entry;

(g) the date of the decision or order that results in an entry under this subsection; and

(h) any other information authorized to be entered by the regulations.

Directories

(2) The Registrar shall maintain one or more directories in which is entered the name of every person who is the holder of a certificate of accreditation identifying the location and class of the veterinary facility

for which the certificate of accreditation is issued, the conditions and limitations attached to the certificate of accreditation, the date of expiry of the certificate of accreditation, every revocation or suspension of a certificate of accreditation and any other information authorized to be entered by the regulations.

Inspection

(3) Any person has the right, during normal business hours, to inspect the registers and directories maintained by the Registrar.

Form of registers and directories

(4) The Registrar may maintain the registers and directories mentioned in subsections (1) and (2) in the form of books or may maintain them in any electronic or other medium that provides a visual display of recorded information. 1989, c. 60, s. 19.

Continuation of memberships

20. Every person who was a member, other than a life member, of the Ontario Veterinary Association immediately before the 4th day of April, 1990 shall be deemed to be the holder of a licence subject to the terms, conditions and limitations that applied to the person's registration, and is a member of the College. 1989, c. 60, s. 20.

Continuation of certificates of accreditation

21. Every certificate of accreditation issued under the *Veterinarians Act*, being chapter 522 of the Revised Statutes of Ontario, 1980, and in force immediately before the 4th day of April, 1990 shall be deemed to be a certificate of accreditation issued under this Act subject to the terms, conditions and limitations that applied to it immediately before the 4th day of April, 1990. 1989, c. 60, s. 21.

Referral of certificate of accreditation

22.—(1) The Registrar may refer a certificate of accreditation to the Accreditation Committee where the Registrar is of the opinion that there is reasonable ground for believing that,

(a) the holder of the certificate of accreditation or the veterinary facility in respect of which the certificate of accreditation was issued has ceased to meet the qualifications, requirements and standards prescribed by the regulations and by the Council for the issuance or renewal of the certificate of accreditation;

(b) the veterinary facility in respect of which the certificate of accreditation was issued is being used or has been used in contravention of a term, condition or limitation of the certificate of accreditation; or

(c) the veterinary facility in respect of which the certificate of accreditation was issued is being used or has been used as a veterinary facility of a class other than the class for which the certificate of accreditation was issued or renewed.

Hearing

(2) The Accreditation Committee shall appoint a time for, give notice of and hold a hearing to determine the allegation in respect of the certificate of accreditation or the holder thereof.

Powers of Accreditation Committee

(3) Where the Accreditation Committee finds that an allegation mentioned in clause (1) (a), (b) or (c) is valid, the Accreditation Committee may, by order,

(a) revoke the certificate of accreditation;

(b) suspend the certificate of accreditation for a stated period not exceeding two years;

(c) suspend the certificate of accreditation pending the demonstration, in such manner as the Committee specifies, of compliance with such standards as are specified by the Committee;

(d) change the class of veterinary facility authorized by the certificate of accreditation; or

(e) impose such conditions and limitations or such further conditions and limitations on the certificate of accreditation as are specified by the Committee,

or any combination thereof.

Procedures   (4) Subsections 28 (5) to (15) and section 29, which relate to proceedings before the Discipline Committee, apply with necessary modifications to proceedings before the Accreditation Committee under subsection (2).

Parties   (5) The College and the holder of the certificate of accreditation in respect of which the hearing is held are parties to the hearing before the Accreditation Committee under subsection (2).

Other proceedings   (6) The jurisdiction of the Discipline Committee is not affected by the commencement of proceedings or the making of an order under this section. 1989, c. 60, s. 22.

Complaints Committee   **23.**—(1) The Complaints Committee shall be composed of not fewer than three and not more than ten persons of whom,

(a) at least one is a member of the Council appointed to the Council by the Lieutenant Governor in Council; and

(b) the others are members of the College, of whom at least one, but not the majority, is a member of the Council.

Eligibility   (2) A member of the Complaints Committee who takes part in the consideration or investigation of a complaint regarding the conduct of a member or former member of the College is not eligible to take part as a member of the Discipline Committee in proceedings before the Discipline Committee in respect of the same conduct of the member or former member of the College.

Quorum   (3) A majority of the members of the Complaints Committee, one of whom is a person appointed to the Council by the Lieutenant Governor in Council, constitutes a quorum. 1989, c. 60, s. 23.

Duties of Complaints Committee   **24.**—(1) The Complaints Committee shall consider and investigate complaints made by members of the public or members of the College regarding the conduct of a member or former member of the College, but no action shall be taken by the Committee under subsection (2) unless,

(a) a written complaint has been filed with the Registrar and the member or former member whose conduct is being investigated has been notified of the complaint and given at least two weeks in which to submit in writing to the Committee any explanations or representations the member or former member may wish to make concerning the matter; and

(b) the Committee has examined or has made every reasonable effort to examine all records and other documents relating to the complaint.

Idem   (2) The Complaints Committee in accordance with the information it receives may,

(a) direct that the matter be referred, in whole or in part, to the Discipline Committee or, for the purposes of section 33, be brought to the attention of the Registrar;

(b) direct that the matter not be referred to the Discipline Committee or brought to the attention of the Registrar under clause (a); or

(c) take such action as it considers appropriate in the circumstances and that is not inconsistent with this Act or the regulations or by-laws.

Decision and reasons   (3) The Complaints Committee shall give its decision in writing to the Registrar and, where the decision is made under clause (2) (b) or (c), its reasons therefor.

Advice   (4) The Complaints Committee may require the member or former member whose conduct was considered or investigated by the Committee to appear before the Committee and the Committee may provide the member or former member with advice in respect of the practice of veterinary medicine. 1989, c. 60, s. 24.

Complaints   **25.**—(1) Where the Complaints Committee has made a disposition of a complaint respecting a member or former member of the College under section 24, the Registrar shall send to the member or former member and to the complainant, by prepaid first class mail, a copy of the written decision made by the Committee including reasons therefor, if any, together with notice advising of the right of review under subsection (2).

Review of complaints   (2) A complainant or the member or former member of the College complained against who is not satisfied with the decision made by the Complaints Committee disposing of a complaint, except a decision to refer a matter to the Discipline Committee or to bring a matter to the attention of the Registrar, may within twenty days of the mailing of the written decision request the Board to review the decision.

Idem   (3) Upon receipt of a request under subsection (2), the Board shall require the Registrar to transmit to the Board within fifteen days of the Board's request a record of the investigation and all such documents and things upon which the decision was based and the Board shall review the decision after giving the complainant an opportunity to state his or her complaint and the member or former member an opportunity to state his or her answer thereto personally, by an agent or in writing.

Closed to the public   (4) Despite the *Statutory Powers Procedure Act*, a review by the Board shall be closed to the public, but if the member or former member whose conduct or actions are the subject-matter of the review requests otherwise by a notice delivered to the Board before the day fixed for the review, the

Board shall conduct the review in public except where the Board is of the opinion that,

    (a) matters involving public security may be disclosed; or

    (b) the possible disclosure of intimate financial or personal matters outweighs the desirability of holding the review in public.

Publication prohibited

(5) Subsections 29 (1), (2) and (3), which relate to proceedings of the Discipline Committee, apply with necessary modifications to a review by the Board under this section. 1989, c. 60, s. 25.

Investigation of complaint by Board

26. Where a complaint respecting a member or former member of the College has not been disposed of by the Complaints Committee within 120 days after the complaint is made, the Board upon application therefor may require the Complaints Committee to make an investigation and, where the investigation of the complaint has not been undertaken, completed and reported on to the Board by the Committee within 120 days after the Board's request, the Board shall undertake such investigation and possesses all the powers of investigation of the Complaints Committee under this Act. 1989, c. 60, s. 26.

Powers of Board after review or investigation of complaint

27.—(1) The Board may, after review or investigation of a complaint under section 25 or 26,

    (a) confirm the decision, if any, made by the Complaints Committee;

    (b) make such recommendations to the Complaints Committee as the Board considers appropriate; or

    (c) require the Complaints Committee to take such action or proceeding as the Committee is authorized to undertake under this Act.

Board quorum

(2) Three members of the Board constitute a quorum for the purposes of an investigation or review of a complaint.

Decision and reasons

(3) The Board shall give its decision and reasons therefor in writing to the complainant and the member of the College complained against. 1989, c. 60, s. 27.

Discipline Committee

28.—(1) The Discipline Committee shall be composed of ten members of the Council of whom two shall be persons appointed to the Council by the Lieutenant Governor in Council.

Quorum and votes

(2) Three members of the Discipline Committee, one of whom is a person appointed to the Council by the Lieutenant Governor in Council, constitute a quorum, and all disciplinary decisions of the Committee require the vote of a majority of the members of the Committee present at the meeting.

Panels

(3) The Discipline Committee may sit in two or more panels simultaneously so long as a quorum of the Committee is present in each panel.

Assignment

(4) The person chairing the Discipline Committee shall assign the members of the Committee to its panels and may change an assignment at any time.

Expiry of member's term of office

(5) Where a proceeding is commenced before the Discipline Committee and the term of office on the Council or on the Committee of a person sitting for the hearing expires or is terminated, other than for cause, before the proceeding has been disposed of but after evidence has been heard, the person shall be deemed to remain a member of the Committee for the purpose of completing the proceeding in the same manner as if the person's term of office had not expired or been terminated.

Disability of member

(6) Where the Discipline Committee commences a hearing and any member thereof becomes unable to continue to act, the remaining members may complete the hearing despite the absence of the member or members and may render a decision as effectually as if all members of the Committee were present throughout the hearing, despite the absence of a quorum of the Committee.

Findings of facts

(7) The findings of fact of the Discipline Committee pursuant to a hearing shall be based exclusively on evidence admissible or matters that may be noticed under sections 15 and 16 of the *Statutory Powers Procedure Act.*

Examination of documentary evidence

(8) A party to a hearing before the Discipline Committee shall be afforded an opportunity to examine before the hearing any written or documentary evidence that will be produced or any report the contents of which will be given in evidence at the hearing.

Delivery of expert witness report

(9) A party to a hearing before the Discipline Committee who intends to call an expert witness at the hearing shall, at least ten days before the commencement of the hearing, deliver to the other party a report, signed by the expert, setting out his or her name, address and qualifications and the substance of his or her proposed testimony.

Exception for expert testimony

(10) An expert witness shall not testify at a hearing before the Discipline Committee unless subsection (9) has been complied with, except,

    (a) with the permission of the Committee;

    (b) with the consent of the other party; or

    (c) to give reply evidence.

Members holding hearing not to have taken part in investigation, etc.

(11) Members of the Discipline Committee holding a hearing shall not have taken part before the hearing in any investigation or consideration of the subject-matter of the hearing other than as a member of the Council or the Executive Committee considering the referral of the matter to the Discipline Committee or at a previous hearing of the Committee, and shall not communicate directly or indirectly in relation to the subject-matter of the hearing with any person or with any party or any party's representative except upon notice to and opportunity for all parties to participate, but the Committee may seek legal advice from an adviser independent from the parties and, in such case, the nature of the advice shall be made known to the parties in order that they may make submissions as to the law. 1989, c. 60, s. 28 (1-11).

Recording of evidence

(12) The oral evidence taken before the Discipline Committee at a hearing shall be recorded and, if so required, copies of a transcript of the oral evidence shall be furnished upon the same terms as in the Ontario Court (General Division). 1989, c. 60, s. 28 (12), *revised.*

Only members at hearing to participate in decision (13) No member of the Discipline Committee shall participate in a decision of the Committee following upon a hearing unless he or she was present throughout the hearing and heard the evidence and argument of the parties.

Release of documentary evidence (14) Documents and things put in evidence at a hearing shall, upon the request of the person who produced them, be released to the person within a reasonable time after the matter in issue has been finally determined.

Practice and procedure (15) The Discipline Committee may determine its own practice and procedure in relation to hearings and may, subject to section 28 of the *Statutory Powers Procedure Act*, make rules governing such practice and procedure and the exercise of its powers in relation thereto that are not inconsistent with this Act and may prescribe such forms as are considered advisable.

Parties (16) The College and the member or former member of the College whose conduct is being investigated are parties to the proceedings before the Discipline Committee. 1989, c. 60, s. 28 (13-16).

Publication prohibited **29.**—(1) No person shall,

(a) take or attempt to take a photograph, motion picture, audio or video recording or other record capable of producing visual or aural representations by any means,

(i) of any person at a hearing of the Discipline Committee,

(ii) of any person entering or leaving a hearing of the Discipline Committee, or

(iii) of any person in the building in which a hearing of the Discipline Committee is held, where there is reasonable ground for believing that the person is there for the purpose of attending the hearing; or

(b) publish, broadcast, reproduce or otherwise disseminate a photograph, motion picture, audio or video recording or record taken in contravention of clause (a).

Exception (2) Subsection (1) does not apply to,

(a) a person unobtrusively making handwritten notes or sketches at a hearing;

(b) a solicitor or party unobtrusively making an audio recording at a hearing that is used only as a substitute for handwritten notes for the purposes of the hearing;

(c) a person taking a photograph, motion picture, audio or video recording or other record with the authorization of the Discipline Committee for any purpose of the hearing; or

(d) a person taking a photograph, motion picture, audio or video recording or other record with the authorization of the Discipline Committee and the consent of the parties and of the witnesses to be recorded, for such educational or instructional purposes as the Committee approves.

Identification prohibited (3) No person shall publish by any means the name of a member or former member of the College who is a party to a hearing by the Discipline Committee or any information which could reasonably serve to identify the member or former member,

(a) unless the member or former member consents to such publication; or

(b) until the Discipline Committee completes the hearing and makes a decision that is required by subsection 19 (1) to be entered in a register.

Exception (4) Despite subsection (3), the Registrar may notify any person who, in the Registrar's opinion, is interested in a Discipline Committee hearing into the conduct of a member or former member of the College of the time and place of the hearing and, in so doing, may identify the member or former member. 1989, c. 60, s. 29.

Reference to Discipline Committee **30.**—(1) The Council or the Executive Committee, by resolution, may direct the Discipline Committee to hold a hearing and determine any allegation of professional misconduct or serious neglect on the part of a member or former member of the College specified in the resolution.

Duties of Discipline Committee (2) The Discipline Committee shall,

(a) when so directed by the Council, the Executive Committee or the Complaints Committee, hear and determine allegations of professional misconduct or serious neglect against a member or former member of the College;

(b) hear and determine matters referred to it under section 37; and

(c) perform such other duties as are assigned to it by the Council.

Professional misconduct (3) A member or former member of the College shall be found guilty of professional misconduct by the Discipline Committee if,

(a) the member or former member has been found guilty of an offence relevant to the suitability to practise veterinary medicine, upon proof of such finding;

(b) the member's or former member's rights or privileges related to the practice of veterinary medicine under an Act of the Parliament of Canada or of the Legislature of Ontario, other than this Act, or the regulations thereunder, have been restricted or withdrawn, unless by the request of the member or former member, upon proof thereof;

(c) there has been a finding of professional misconduct or serious neglect, or a like finding, against the member or former member by a veterinary authority in another jurisdiction, upon proof of such finding; or

(d) the member or former member has been guilty in the opinion of the Committee of professional misconduct as defined in the regulations.

Serious neglect (4) A member or former member of the College shall be found guilty of serious neglect by the Discipline Committee if the member or former member has displayed in his or her professional care of an animal a lack of knowledge, skill or judgment or disregard for the welfare of the animal of a nature or to an extent that demonstrates the member or former member is unfit to engage in the practice of veterinary medicine or is fit to engage in the practice of veterinary medicine only subject to the conditions and limitations imposed by the Discipline Committee.

Powers of Discipline Committee

(5) Where the Discipline Committee finds a member or former member of the College guilty of professional misconduct or serious neglect, it may by order,

(a) revoke the licence of the member;

(b) withdraw recognition of the specialist status of the member;

(c) suspend the licence of the member or suspend recognition of the specialist status of the member, or both, for a stated period or pending the demonstration of such facts as are specified by the Committee;

(d) impose such conditions and limitations upon the licence of the member for such period of time as is specified by the Committee or pending the demonstration of such facts as are specified by the Committee;

(e) impose such fine as the Committee considers appropriate, to a maximum of $5,000, to be paid by the member or former member to the Treasurer of Ontario for payment into the Consolidated Revenue Fund;

(f) reprimand the member or former member;

(g) direct that the imposition of a penalty be suspended or postponed for such period and upon such terms as the Committee designates,

or any combination thereof.

Costs

(6) Where the Discipline Committee is of the opinion that the commencement of the proceedings was unwarranted, the Committee shall order that the College reimburse the member or former member of the College for his or her costs or such portion thereof as the Committee fixes.

Register entries

(7) Where the Discipline Committee imposes a fine or reprimands a member or former member, the Committee may direct that the fact and amount of the fine or the fact of the reprimand not be entered in a register required to be kept under subsection 19 (1). 1989, c. 60, s. 30.

Publication and service of decision of Discipline Committee

31.—(1) Where the Discipline Committee finds a member or former member of the College guilty of professional misconduct or serious neglect,

(a) the Registrar shall publish the finding, with or without the reasons therefor, in a publication of the College; and

(b) the Registrar shall serve a copy of the decision upon the person, if any, complaining in respect of the conduct or actions of the member or former member.

When name is published

(2) If the finding of the Discipline Committee is required by subsection 19 (1) to be recorded in a register, the Registrar shall include the name of the member or former member in the publication required under clause (1) (a).

When name is not published

(3) If the Discipline Committee directs that no entry be made in a register, the Registrar shall not include the name of the member or former member in the publication required under clause (1) (a). 1989, c. 60, s. 31.

Stay of decision on appeal, serious neglect

32.—(1) Where the Discipline Committee revokes or suspends a licence, withdraws or suspends recognition of specialist status or imposes conditions or limitations upon a licence on the ground of serious neglect, the decision takes effect immediately even if an appeal is taken from the decision, unless the court to which the appeal is taken otherwise orders.

Stay of decision on appeal, professional misconduct

(2) Where the Discipline Committee revokes or suspends a licence, withdraws or suspends recognition of specialist status or imposes conditions or limitations upon a licence on the ground of professional misconduct, the order does not take effect until the time for appeal from the order has expired without an appeal being taken or, if taken, the appeal has been disposed of or abandoned. 1989, c. 60, s. 32.

Definition

33.—(1) In this section, "board of inquiry" means a board of inquiry appointed by the Executive Committee under subsection (2).

Board of inquiry

(2) Where the Registrar receives information leading the Registrar to believe that a member of the College may be impaired, the Registrar shall make such inquiry as he or she considers appropriate and report to the Executive Committee which may, upon notice to the member of the College, appoint a board of inquiry composed of at least two members of the College and one member of the Council appointed thereto by the Lieutenant Governor in Council.

Examination

(3) The board of inquiry shall make such inquiries as it considers appropriate and may require the member of the College to submit to physical and mental examinations by such qualified persons as the board of inquiry designates, but not to more than one examination in each area of medical specialty and if the member of the College refuses or fails to submit to such examinations, the board of inquiry may order that the member's licence be suspended until he or she complies.

Hearing by Registration Committee

(4) The board of inquiry shall report its findings to the Executive Committee and deliver a copy thereof and a copy of any report obtained under subsection (3) to the member of the College about whom the report is made and if, in the opinion of the Executive Committee, the evidence so warrants, the Executive Committee shall refer the matter to the Registration Committee to hold a hearing and may suspend the member's licence until the determination of whether or not the member is impaired becomes final.

Parties

(5) The College, the member of the College being investigated and any other person specified by the Registration Committee are parties to a hearing before the Registration Committee under this section.

Medical evidence

(6) A legally qualified medical practitioner is not compellable to produce at the hearing his or her case histories, notes or any other records constituting medical evidence but, when required to give evidence, shall prepare a report containing the medical facts, findings, conclusions and treatment.

Idem

(7) The report required under subsection (6) is receivable in evidence without proof of its making or of the signature of the legally qualified medical practitioner making the report but a party who is not tendering the report as evidence has the right to summon and cross-examine the medical practitioner on the contents of the report.

Powers of Registration Committee

(8) The Registration Committee shall, after the hearing,

(a) make a finding as to whether or not the member of the College is impaired; and

(b) where the member of the College is found to be impaired, by order,

(i) revoke the member's licence,

(ii) suspend the member's licence either indefinitely or pending the demonstration of such facts as the Committee specifies, or

(iii) impose such conditions and limitations upon the member's licence as the Committee considers appropriate.

Procedures

(9) Subsections 28 (5) to (15) and 29 (1), (2) and (3), which relate to proceedings of the Discipline Committee, apply with necessary modifications to proceedings of the Registration Committee under this section.

Closed to the public

(10) Despite the *Statutory Powers Procedure Act*, a hearing by the Registration Committee under this section shall be closed to the public but, if the member of the College who is the subject-matter of the hearing requests otherwise by a notice delivered to the Registration Committee before the day fixed for the hearing, the Registration Committee shall conduct the hearing in public except where,

(a) matters involving public security may be disclosed; or

(b) the possible disclosure of intimate financial or personal matters outweighs the desirability of holding the hearing in public.

Continuing jurisdiction over former member

(11) Subsections (1) to (10) apply with necessary modifications to an inquiry or hearing into whether or not a former member of the College was impaired when he or she was a member of the College, and for such purposes the board of inquiry or Registration Committee, as the case may be, may provide that the revocation or suspension of a licence or the imposition of conditions or limitations upon a licence take effect at the same time as or immediately after an existing revocation or suspension. 1989, c. 60, s. 33.

Stay of decision on appeal

34. Where the Registration Committee revokes, suspends or imposes conditions or limitations upon the licence of a member of the College on the ground that the member

is impaired, the decision takes effect immediately even if an appeal is taken from the decision, unless the court to which the appeal is taken otherwise orders. 1989, c. 60, s. 34.

Appeal to court

35.—(1) A party to,

(a) a proceeding before the Discipline Committee under section 30;

(b) a proceeding before the Registration Committee under section 33;

(c) a proceeding before the Accreditation Committee under section 22;

(d) a hearing by the Board in respect of a proposal by the Registration Committee related to the issuance of a licence or the imposition of conditions or limitations on a licence; or

(e) a hearing by the Board in respect of a proposal by the Accreditation Committee related to the issuance or renewal of a certificate of accreditation or the imposition of conditions or limitations on a certificate of accreditation,

may appeal to the Divisional Court from the decision or order of the committee or the Board.

Certified copy of record

(2) Upon the request of a party desiring to appeal to the Divisional Court and upon payment of a reasonable administrative fee therefor, the Registrar or the Executive Secretary of the Board, as the case requires, shall furnish the party with a certified copy of the record of the proceedings.

Powers of court on appeal

(3) An appeal under this section may be made on questions of law or fact or both and the court may affirm or may rescind the decision of the Board or the committee appealed from and may exercise all powers of the Board or the committee appealed from to take any action which the Board or the committee appealed from may take and as the court considers proper, and for such purposes the court may substitute its opinion for that of the Board or the committee appealed from or the court may refer the matter back to the Board or the committee appealed from for rehearing, in whole or in part, in accordance with such directions as the court considers proper. 1989, c. 60, s. 35.

Registrar's investigation

36.—(1) Where the Registrar believes on reasonable ground that a member or former member of the College has committed an act of professional misconduct or serious neglect or that there is cause to refuse to issue or renew or to suspend or revoke a certificate of accreditation, the Registrar, with the approval of the Executive Committee, by order may appoint one or more persons to investigate whether such act has occurred or whether there is such cause, and the person or persons appointed shall report the results of the investigation to the Registrar.

Powers of investigator

(2) For purposes relevant to the subject-matter of an investigation under this section, a person appointed to make an investigation may inquire into and examine the practice of the member or former member in respect of whom the investigation is being made and may, upon production of his or her appointment, enter at any reasonable time the business premises of the member or former member, make reasonable inquiries of any

person and examine documents and things relevant to the subject-matter of the investigation.

Co-operation with investigator (3) Every member and former member of the College shall co-operate fully with a person appointed to make an investigation into his or her practice.

Order by justice of the peace (4) Where a justice of the peace is satisfied on evidence upon oath that the Registrar had grounds for appointing and by order has appointed one or more persons to make an investigation, the justice may, whether or not an investigation has been made or attempted under subsection (2), issue a warrant authorizing the person or persons making the investigation and named in the warrant, to enter any premises in which the member or former member of the College in respect of whom the investigation is being made has engaged in the practice of veterinary medicine or maintained records, to search for any documents or things relevant to the subject-matter of the investigation.

Authority to use force (5) A warrant issued under subsection (4) authorizes the person or persons named in the warrant to carry out the warrant by force if necessary and together with such police officers as are called upon for assistance.

Execution of warrant (6) A warrant issued under subsection (4) shall specify the hours and days during which it may be executed.

Expiry of warrant (7) A warrant issued under subsection (4) shall state the date on which it expires, which shall be a date not later than fifteen days after the warrant is issued.

Application without notice (8) A justice of the peace may receive and consider an application for a warrant under subsection (4) without notice to and in the absence of the member or former member of the College whose practice is being investigated.

Removal of documents and things (9) Any person making an investigation under this section may, upon giving a receipt therefor, remove any documents or things examined under this section relating to the member or former member whose practice is being investigated and to the subject-matter of the investigation for the purpose of making copies or extracts and shall promptly return such documents or things to the member or former member whose practice is being investigated.

Admissibility of copies (10) Any copy or extract made as provided in subsection (9) and certified to be a true copy or extract by the person who made it is admissible in evidence to the same extent as, and has the same evidentiary value as, the document or thing of which it is a copy or extract.

Report of Registrar (11) The Registrar shall report the results of the investigation to the Council or such committee as the Registrar considers appropriate. 1989, c. 60, s. 36.

Application for licence after revocation **37.**—(1) A person whose licence has been revoked for cause under this Act, or whose registration has been cancelled for cause under a predecessor of this Act, may apply in writing to the Registrar for the issuance of a licence, but the application shall not be made sooner than two years after the revocation or cancellation or one year after any prior application for issuance of the licence.

Removal of suspension (2) A person whose licence has been suspended for cause under this Act, or whose registration has been suspended for cause under a predecessor of this Act, for more than one year or for other than a specific period, may apply in writing to the Registrar for the removal of the suspension, but the application shall not be made sooner than one year after the commencement of the suspension or one year after any prior application for the removal of the suspension.

Variation of licence restrictions (3) A person to whose licence terms, conditions or limitations have been attached for cause under this Act, or under a predecessor of this Act, may apply in writing to the Registrar for removal or alteration of the terms, conditions or limitations, but the application shall not be made sooner than one year after the commencement of the terms, conditions or limitations or one year after any prior application for removal or alteration of the terms, conditions or limitations.

Exemptions (4) Subsection (3) does not apply to a person whose licence is the subject of conditions or limitations imposed as a result of a proposal or decision of the Registration Committee under clause 14 (6) (c).

Referral to committee (5) The Registrar shall refer an application under subsection (1), (2) or (3) to the committee that ordered the revocation, suspension, condition or limitation, as the case may be, and the committee shall hold a hearing respecting the application.

Idem, orders under predecessor Act (6) Where the council of the Ontario Veterinary Association ordered the cancellation, suspension, term or condition under a predecessor of this Act, the Registrar shall refer the application under subsection (1), (2) or (3) to the committee which, under this Act, would have jurisdiction over the subject-matter that resulted in the cancellation, suspension, term or condition and the committee shall hold a hearing respecting the application.

Hearing by Registration Committee (7) Subsections 28 (5) to (15) and 29 (1), (2) and (3), which relate to hearings by the Discipline Committee, and subsection 33 (10), which relates to hearings by the Registration Committee into whether or not a member is impaired, apply with necessary modifications to proceedings of the Registration Committee under this section.

Hearing by Discipline Committee (8) The provisions of this Act which relate to proceedings of the Discipline Committee apply to proceedings of the Discipline Committee under this section.

Parties (9) The applicant and the College are parties to a hearing under subsection (5) or (6).

Powers of committee (10) The committee shall, after the hearing under subsection (5) or (6), report its decision and reasons to the parties and direct the Registrar,

(a) to issue the licence;

(b) to refuse to issue the licence;

(c) to issue the licence subject to the conditions and limitations the committee specifies;

(d) to remove the suspension of the licence;

(e) to refuse to remove the suspension of the licence;

(f) to remove or alter any of the terms, conditions or limitations attached to the licence; or

(g) to refuse to remove or alter any of the terms, conditions or limitations attached to the licence. 1989, c. 60, s. 37.

Confiden-
tiality

38.—(1) Every person engaged in the administration of this Act, including any person making an investigation under section 36, shall preserve secrecy with respect to all matters that come to his or her knowledge in the course of his or her duties, employment, examination, review or investigation and shall not communicate any such matters to any other person except,

(a) as may be permitted by the regulations or required in connection with the administration of this Act and the regulations and by-laws, or any proceeding under this Act or the regulations;

(b) to his or her counsel; or

(c) with the consent of the person to whom the information relates.

Testimony in
civil action

(2) No person to whom subsection (1) applies shall be required to give testimony or to produce any document or thing in any action or proceeding with regard to information obtained in the course of his or her duties, employment, examination, review or investigation except in a proceeding under this Act or the regulations.

Board

(3) For the purposes of subsections (1) and (2), the Board, each member of the Board and each member of the staff of the Board shall be deemed to be a person engaged in the administration of this Act. 1989, c. 60, s. 38.

Order
directing
compliance

39.—(1) Where it appears to the College that any person does not comply with any provision of this Act or the regulations, despite the imposition of any penalty in respect of such non-compliance and in addition to any other rights it may have, the College may apply to a judge of the Ontario Court (General Division) for an order directing the person to comply with the provision, and upon the application the judge may make the order or such other order as the judge thinks fit. 1989, c. 60, s. 39 (1), *revised.*

Appeal

(2) An appeal lies to the Divisional Court from an order made under subsection (1). 1989, c. 60, s. 39 (2).

Penalties

40.—(1) Every person who contravenes section 11 is guilty of an offence and on conviction is liable for the first offence to a fine of not more than $15,000 and for each subsequent offence to a fine of not more than $30,000.

Idem, use of
titles

(2) Every person who is not a holder of a licence and who,

(a) uses the title "veterinarian", "vétérinaire", or "veterinary surgeon", "chirurgien vétérinaire" or an abbreviation or variation thereof as an occupational or business designation; or

(b) uses a term, title or description that will lead to the belief that the person may engage in the practice of veterinary medicine,

is guilty of an offence and on conviction is liable for the first offence to a fine of not more than $5,000 and for each subsequent offence to a fine of not more than $15,000.

Idem, publi-
cation

(3) Every person who contravenes subsection 29 (1) or (3) is guilty of an offence and on conviction is liable to a fine of not more than $10,000 and for each subsequent offence to a fine of not more than $20,000.

Corporation

(4) Where a corporation is convicted of an offence under subsection (1), (2) or (3), the maximum fine that may be imposed is $25,000 on a first conviction and $50,000 on each subsequent conviction and not as provided in subsection (1), (2) or (3).

Offence,
director,
officer, etc.,
of corpora-
tion

(5) Where a corporation is convicted of an offence under subsection (1), (2) or (3),

(a) each director of the corporation; and

(b) each officer, employee or agent of the corporation who was in whole or in part responsible for the conduct of that part of the business of the corporation that gave rise to the offence,

is guilty of an offence unless he or she proves, on the balance of probabilities, that he or she took all reasonable care to prevent the commission of the offence.

Idem,
penalty

(6) Every person convicted of an offence under subsection (5) is liable on conviction to a fine of not more than $15,000 on a first conviction and not more than $30,000 on each subsequent conviction.

Limitation

(7) Proceedings shall not be commenced in respect of an offence under subsection (1), (2), (3) or (5) after two years after the date on which the offence was, or is alleged to have been, committed. 1989, c. 60, s. 40.

Falsification
of docu-
ments

41.—(1) Any person who makes or causes to be made a wilful falsification in a matter relating to a register or directory or issues a false licence, certificate of accreditation or document with respect to the issuance of a licence or certificate of accreditation is guilty of an offence and on conviction is liable to a fine of not more than $5,000.

Offences for
false repre-
sentation

(2) Every person who wilfully procures or attempts to procure the issuance of a licence or a certificate of accreditation under this Act by knowingly making a false representation or declaration or by making a fraudulent representation or declaration, either orally or in writing, is guilty of an offence and on conviction is liable to a fine of not more than $5,000.

Limitation
period

(3) Proceedings to obtain a conviction for an offence under subsection (1) or (2) shall not be commenced after the expiration of one year after the date on which the offence was, or is alleged to have been, committed. 1989, c. 60, s. 41.

Onus of proof respecting licensing

42. Where licensing or acting under and in accordance with a certificate of accreditation under this Act is required to permit the lawful doing of an act or thing, if in any prosecution it is proven that the defendant has done the act or thing, the burden of proving that he or she was so licensed or that he or she acted under and in accordance with a certificate of accreditation under this Act rests upon the defendant. 1989, c. 60, s. 42.

Service of notice or document

43.—(1) A notice or document under this Act or the regulations is sufficiently given, served or delivered if delivered personally or by mail.

Idem

(2) Where a notice or document under this Act or the regulations is sent to a person by mail addressed to the person at the last address of the person in the records of the College, there is a rebuttable presumption that the notice or document is delivered to the person on the fifth day after the day of mailing. 1989, c. 60, s. 43.

Registrar's certificate as evidence

44. Any statement containing information from the records required to be kept by the Registrar under this Act and purporting to be certified by the Registrar under the seal of the College is admissible in evidence in all courts and tribunals as proof, in the absence of evidence to the contrary, of the facts stated therein without proof of the appointment or signature of the Registrar and without proof of the seal. 1989, c. 60, s. 44.

Immunity

45.—(1) No action or other proceeding for damages shall be instituted against the Board, the College, the Council, a committee of the College or a member of the Board, the Council or a committee of the College, or an officer, employee, agent or appointee of the Board or of the College for any act done in good faith in the performance or intended performance of a duty or in the exercise or the intended exercise of a power under this Act, a regulation or a by-law, or for any neglect or default in the performance or exercise in good faith of such duty or power.

Councillor indemnified in suits respecting duties of office

(2) Every member of the Council or a committee of the College and every officer and employee of the College, and their heirs, executors and administrators, and estate and effects, respectively, shall from time to time and at all times, be indemnified and saved harmless out of the funds of the College, from and against,

(a) all costs, charges and expenses whatsoever that he or she sustains or incurs in or about any action or proceeding brought or commenced against him or her in respect of any act, deed, matter or thing whatsoever, made, done or permitted by him or her, in or about the execution of the duties of his or her office; and

(b) all other costs, charges and expenses that he or she sustains or incurs in or about or in relation to the affairs thereof,

except such costs, charges or expenses as are occasioned by his or her own wilful neglect or default. 1989, c. 60, s. 45.

Limitation of action

46. Proceedings shall not be commenced against a member of the College for damages arising from the provision of a service that is within the practice of veterinary medicine after one year from the date when the person commencing the action knew or ought to have known the fact or facts upon which the allegations are based. 1989, c. 60, s. 46.

Corporations Act applies in part

47.—(1) The *Corporations Act* does not apply in respect of the College except for the following sections of that Act which apply with necessary modifications in respect of the College:

1. Section 81 (liability for wages).

2. Section 94 (auditors) and, for the purpose, the Minister shall be deemed to be the Minister referred to in the section.

3. Subsection 95 (1) (auditor's qualifications) and, for the purpose, the subsection shall be deemed not to include,

   i. the exception as provided in subsection 95 (2), and

   ii. the reference to an affiliated company.

4. Section 96 (auditor's functions).

5. Subsection 97 (1), exclusive of clause 97 (1) (b), (auditor's report) and, for the purpose, the College shall be deemed to be a private company.

6. Subsection 97 (2) (designation of statements).

7. Subsection 97 (3) (auditor's report).

8. Section 122 (liability of members).

9. Section 276 (holding of land) and, for the purpose, the Minister shall be deemed to be the Minister referred to in the section.

10. Section 280 (making contracts).

11. Section 281 (power of attorney).

12. Section 282 (authentication of documents) except in respect of information from the records required to be kept by the Registrar.

13. Section 292 (validity of acts of directors).

14. Section 293 (annual meetings).

15. Section 297 (directions by a court as to holding a meeting).

16. Section 299 (minutes of meetings).

17. Section 302 (books of account).

18. Section 303 (untrue entries) and, for the purpose, the section shall be deemed not to refer to section 41 of that Act.

19. Section 304 (place of keeping and inspection of records) and, for the purpose,

    i. the section shall be deemed not to refer to sections 41 (register of transfers) and 43 (registers of transfers) of that Act, and

    ii. the Minister shall be deemed to be the Minister referred to in the section.

20. Section 305 (inspection of records) and, for the purpose, the section shall be deemed not to refer to creditors and to refer to section 41 of that Act.

21. Section 310 (investigations and audits).

22. Section 329 (appeals).

23. Section 330 (untrue statements) and, for the purpose,

    i. the section shall be deemed not to refer to regulations made under that Act, and

    ii. the Minister shall be deemed to be the Minister referred to in the section and the Deputy Minister of the Ministry presided over by the Minister under this Act shall be deemed to be the Deputy Minister referred to in the section.

24. Section 332 (orders by court) and, for the purpose, the section shall be deemed not to refer to creditors. 1989, c. 60, s. 47 (1), *revised*.

Interpretation

(2) For the purposes of subsection (1), a member of the College shall be deemed to be a shareholder and a member of the Council shall be deemed to be a director.

Corporate information

(3) The *Corporations Information Act* does not apply in respect of the College. 1989, c. 60, s. 47 (2, 3).

Interpretation

48. Any reference in any Act or regulation to a veterinarian as a member of the Ontario Veterinary Association under the *Veterinarians Act* being chapter 522 of the Revised Statutes of Ontario, 1980, shall be deemed to be a reference to a member of the College under this Act. 1989, c. 60, s. 48 (2), *revised*.

APPENDIX G

Regulations Under the Veterinarians Act (Ontario)

REGULATION 1093

GENERAL

DEFINITIONS

1. In this Regulation,

"auxiliary" means a person involved in a member's practice of veterinary medicine other than another member;

"member" means a member of the College. R.R.O. 1990, Reg. 1093, s. 1.

PART I
REGISTRATION AND ACCREDITATION

2. In this Part,

"acceptable unaccredited veterinary school" means a veterinary school, other than an accredited veterinary school, that at the time of an applicant's graduation,

(a) provides an undergraduate program of veterinary medical education leading to a basic degree that includes at least 125 weeks of instruction scheduled over a minimum of thirty-two months, and

(b) is listed in the World Directory of Veterinary Schools last published by the World Health Organization or is classified as "AVMA—listed" in the Directory of Veterinary Colleges of the World last published by the American Veterinary Medical Association;

"accredited veterinary school" means a veterinary school that, at the time of an applicant's graduation, is accredited by the Council on Education of the American Veterinary Medical Association;

"basic degree" means a Doctor of Veterinary Medicine or an equivalent degree in veterinary medicine;

"companion animal" does not include a horse;

"local examination" means an examination approved by the Registration Committee on legal and ethical aspects of veterinary practice in Ontario including reportable diseases;

"major surgery" means surgery,

(a) in which bone, viscera or an extensive area of subcutaneous tissue is exposed, or

(b) the failure of which would endanger the life or organ function of the animal. R.R.O. 1990, Reg. 1093, s. 2.

3.—(1) The requirements for the issuing of any licence are that the applicant,

(a) is a Canadian citizen or permanent resident or has another status under the *Immigration Act* (Canada) consistent with the class of licence for which application is made;

(b) has completed the Test of English as a Foreign Language with a minimum score of 550 and the Test of Spoken English with a minimum score of 200 or has successfully completed tests acceptable to the College of the applicant's ability to speak and write in French with scores that reflect a competence that is at least equivalent to the scores required in English;

(c) completes an application for the class of licence for which application is made on a form provided by the Registrar;

(d) if the applicant has previously practised veterinary medicine, provides evidence that there has been no finding of, and that there is no current proceeding involving an allegation of, professional misconduct, gross neglect or impairment;

(e) provides a declaration affirming that there has been no finding of guilt of, and that there is no charge pending involving an allegation of, an offence relevant to the applicant's suitability to practise veterinary medicine;

(f) pays the relevant examination fee, application fee, licence fee, and annual membership fee as set out in the Schedule;

(g) meets the requirements for the class of licence for which application is made; and

(h) submits in person to the Registrar his or her original degree in veterinary medicine and documentation proving his or her identity.

(2) Clause (1) (b) does not apply if the primary and secondary education of the applicant was conducted in English or French or if the undergraduate veterinary education of the applicant was conducted in English or French.

(3) Clause (1) (h) does not apply to an applicant who is a graduate of an accredited veterinary school in Canada or who applies for a short-term licence. R.R.O. 1990, Reg. 1093, s. 3.

4.—(1) A restricted licence is a licence with conditions or limitations imposed by a committee under the Act or by the Council under a predecessor of that Act.

(2) A holder of a restricted licence may practise veterinary medicine only in accordance with the conditions of the licence. R.R.O. 1990, Reg. 1093, s. 4.

5.—(1) The requirements for the issuing of a general licence are that the applicant,

(a) has earned a basic degree from an accredited veterinary school or an acceptable unaccredited veterinary school;

(b) has obtained a score higher than 1.5 standard deviations below the mean on both parts of the national board examination for veterinary medical licensing of the National Board Examination Committee of the American Veterinary Medical Association, including the clinical competency test;

(b.1) despite clause (b), has obtained a passing mark on both parts of the national board examination for veterinary medical licensing of the National Board Examination Committee of the American Veterinary Medical Association, including the clinical competency test, if the examinations are taken on or after the 1st day of December, 1992;

(c) has successfully completed the local examination; and

(d) if a graduate of an acceptable unaccredited veterinary school, after compliance with clause (b) or (b.1), has successfully completed the clinical proficiency examination of the National Examining Board of the Canadian Veterinary Medical Association administered through an accredited veterinary school. R.R.O. 1990, Reg. 1093, s. 5 (1); O. Reg. 407/92, s. 1.

(2) Despite subsection (1), a member who has surrendered a general licence and been issued an educational licence immediately thereafter shall be deemed to have the requirements for the issuing of a general licence for two months after the termination of the educational licence. R.R.O. 1990, Reg. 1093, s. 5 (2).

6.—(1) The requirements for the issuing of an academic licence are that the applicant,

(a) has a basic degree from an accredited veterinary school or an acceptable unaccredited veterinary school;

(b) has a full-time teaching or research appointment of professorial rank in the Ontario Veterinary College of the University of Guelph with full payment at salary of rank paid by the University; and

(c) has successfully completed the local examination.

(2) A holder of an academic licence may engage in the practice of veterinary medicine only in the department in which he or she holds a professorial appointment and to the extent required by that appointment.

(3) An academic licence terminates when the licensee ceases to hold an appointment in accordance with clause (1) (b). R.R.O. 1990, Reg. 1093, s. 6.

7.—(1) The requirements for the issuing of a public service licence are that the applicant,

(a) has earned a basic degree from an accredited veterinary school or an acceptable unaccredited veterinary school; and

(b) is employed as a veterinarian by the Crown in right of Canada. R.R.O. 1990, Reg. 1093, s. 7 (1); O. Reg. 308/91, s. 1 (1).

(2) A holder of a public service licence may engage in the practice of veterinary medicine only in the course of employment as a veterinarian by the Crown in right of Canada. R.R.O. 1990, Reg. 1093, s. 7 (2); O. Reg. 308/91, s. 1 (2).

(3) A public service licence terminates when the licensee ceases to be employed as a veterinarian by the Crown in right of Canada. R.R.O. 1990, Reg. 1093, s. 7 (3); O. Reg. 308/91, s. 1 (3).

8.—(1) The requirements for the issuing of a short-term licence are that the applicant,

(a) has earned a basic degree from an accredited veterinary school or an acceptable unaccredited veterinary school;

(b) provides a document from a member holding a general licence without conditions that evidences the member's undertaking to supervise the applicant and to be responsible for continuing after the licensee leaves Ontario any veterinary care started in Ontario by the licensee; and

(c) is appointed by the Ontario Veterinary College of the University of Guelph, a regional academy of veterinary medicine in Ontario or a recognized group of members with special veterinary interest, or has the consent of the College, to perform specific veterinary services solely for a short-term, special purpose.

(2) A holder of a short-term licence may engage in the practice of veterinary medicine only under the supervision of the member whose undertaking has been given under clause (1) (b) and to the extent required by the appointment or consent under clause (1) (c).

(3) A short-term licence terminates on the earliest of,

(a) the day the appointment or consent under clause (1) (c) is terminated;

(b) the day the licensee leaves Ontario; and

(c) thirty days after the licence is issued. R.R.O. 1990, Reg. 1093, s. 8.

9.—(1) The requirements for the issuing of an educational licence are that the applicant,

(a) has earned a basic degree from an accredited veterinary school or an acceptable unaccredited veterinary school; and

(b) is enrolled in a program of postgraduate veterinary education provided by the Ontario Veterinary College of the University of Guelph.

(2) The holder of an educational licence,

(a) may engage in the practice of veterinary medicine only as required by the program of education in which the licensee is enrolled and only under the supervision of a full-time employee of the University of Guelph who holds a general licence or an academic licence; and

(b) may receive remuneration for veterinary services only in the form of a fixed salary or stipend.

(3) An educational licence terminates when the licensee ceases to be enrolled in a program of postgraduate veterinary education provided by the Ontario Veterinary College of the University of Guelph. R.R.O. 1990, Reg. 1093, s. 9.

10. The requirements for the issuing or renewing of any certificate of accreditation are that the veterinary facility meets the standards established under subsection 8 (1) of the Act for the class of certificate of accreditation for which application is made and the applicant,

(a) submits to the College an application in a form provided by the Registrar;

(b) is the owner of, or a partner in, the practice conducted on or from the facility that is the subject of application, or submits to the College the written authority of the owners or partners of that practice to provide the undertaking required under clause (c);

(c) provides a written undertaking to be responsible for the facility on a form provided by the Registrar;

(d) holds a general licence or a restricted licence the conditions of which are consistent with the conditions of the certificate of accreditation; and

(e) pays the inspection fee set out in the Schedule. R.R.O. 1990, Reg. 1093, s. 10.

11. It is a condition of a certificate of accreditation that the designation of a veterinary facility described in Column A of the Table contains one of the appropriate terms set out in Column B of the Table:

TABLE

	COLUMN A	COLUMN B
1.	Companion animal hospital	Clinic, Hospital or Services
2.	Companion animal office	Office or Services
3.	Companion animal mobile office	Mobile Office or Mobile Services
4.	Companion animal mobile	Mobile, Mobile Services or House Call Services
5.	Companion animal emergency clinic	Emergency Clinic or Emergency Hospital
6.	Companion animal spay-neuter clinic	Spay-Neuter Clinic

	COLUMN A	COLUMN B
7.	Food-producing animal hospital	Clinic, Hospital or Services
8.	Food-producing animal mobile	Mobile, Services or Mobile Services
9.	Equine clinic	Clinic, Hospital or Services
10.	Equine mobile	Mobile, Services or Mobile Services
10.1	Equine Emergency mobile	Emergency Mobile, Emergency Services or Emergency Mobile Services
11.	Poultry service	Clinic or Services

R.R.O. 1990, Reg. 1093, s. 11; O. Reg. 407/92, s. 2.

12.—(1) Subject to subsection (2), a certificate of accreditation expires,

(a) in the case of accreditation following the correction of deficiencies found in an inspection, three years after the certificate of accreditation was issued or renewed; and

(b) in the case of accreditation based upon an inspection in which no deficiencies were found, five years after the certificate of accreditation was issued or renewed.

(2) A certificate of accreditation expires before the period described in subsection (1) if,

(a) a stationary veterinary facility, or a stationary element of a facility with a mobile element, is relocated; or

(b) no member meets the requirements in clauses 10 (a), (b), (c) and (d) in respect of the veterinary facility. R.R.O. 1990, Reg. 1093, s. 12.

13. Every member practising in or from a facility, other than a companion animal mobile, food-producing animal mobile equine mobile or equine emergency mobile, shall ensure that the certificate of accreditation is displayed conspicuously in the facility so that clients can read it easily. R.R.O. 1990, Reg. 1093, s. 13; O. Reg. 407/92, s. 3.

14.—(1) A certificate of accreditation for a companion animal hospital, office, mobile office, mobile, emergency clinic or spay-neuter clinic limits the veterinary practice in or from the facility to the treatment of companion animals.

(2) A certificate of accreditation for a food-producing animal hospital or mobile limits the veterinary practice in or from the facility to the treatment of food-producing animals and horses. R.R.O. 1990, Reg. 1093, s. 14 (1, 2).

(3) A certificate of accreditation for an equine clinic mobile or emergency mobile limits the veterinary practice in or from the facility to the treatment of horses. R.R.O. 1990, Reg. 1093, s. 14 (3); O. Reg. 407/92, s. 4 (1).

(4) A certificate of accreditation for a poultry service limits the veterinary practice in or from the facility to the treatment of poultry.

(5) It is a condition of a certificate of accreditation for a companion animal hospital that the veterinary services provided in or from the facility do not include radiology, major surgery, overnight confinement or, except for observation and continuing care on the day of treatment, hospitalization.

(6) It is a condition of a certificate of accreditation for a companion animal mobile office that the veterinary services provided in or from the facility do not include radiology, major surgery, overnight confinement or hospitalization.

(7) A certificate of accreditation for a companion animal mobile limits the veterinary services provided from the facility to,

(a) assessments;

(b) vaccinations;

(c) tranquilization, sedation or local anaesthesia;

(d) surgical repair of simple wounds for which general anaesthesia is not necessary;

(e) treatment of abscesses for which general anaesthesia is not necessary;

(f) tail docks and dewclaw removals on animals less than one week of age;

(g) nail clipping;

(h) expression of anal glands;

(i) cleansing and treatment of ear conditions for which general anaesthesia is not necessary;

(j) minor dental work for which general anaesthesia is not necessary;

(k) ophthalmic examinations and simple ocular procedures;

(l) collection for screening analysis of blood, skin scrapings, urine and feces;

(m) bandaging;

(n) euthanasia;

(o) emergency care pending transport to a companion animal hospital;

(p) prescribing and dispensing drugs;

(q) collection of semen;

(r) artificial insemination; and

(s) breeding supervision.

(8) It is a condition of a certificate of accreditation for a companion animal emergency clinic that a member is actually on duty in the facility and available for service with reasonable promptness,

(a) every weekday from at least 7 p.m. to 9 a.m. the following day;

(b) every weekend from at least 7 p.m. Friday to 9 a.m. the following Monday; and

(c) every statutory holiday from at least 7 p.m. the day before the holiday to 9 a.m. the day following the holiday.

(9) A certificate of accreditation for a companion animal spay-neuter clinic limits the veterinary services provided in or from the facility to spay and neuter procedures, including the pre-, intra- and post-operative management usually associated with those procedures. R.R.O. 1990, Reg. 1093, s. 14 (4–9).

(10) The following are conditions of a certificate of accreditation for an equine emergency mobile:

1. A member shall be on duty and available for service with reasonable promptness,

   i. every weekend from 7 p.m. on Friday to 9 a.m. on the following Monday, and

   ii. every statutory holiday from 7 p.m. on the day before the holiday to 9 a.m. on the day following the holiday.

2. The holder of the certificate shall ensure that clients are directed to an alternate facility by answering machine or answering service when no member is on duty in the facility. O. Reg. 407/92, s. 4 (2).

15.—(1) The Council may by by-law establish a category of membership for retired members and may,

(a) designate the name by which the category is to be known; and

(b) establish the criteria for membership in the category.

(2) Retired members are entitled to receive the general mailings of the College and notice of meetings and may speak at meetings but are not eligible to vote on any matter.

(3) A retired member may not hold a veterinary licence and may not practise veterinary medicine or hold himself or herself out as engaging in the practice of veterinary medicine. R.R.O. 1990, Reg. 1093, s. 15.

16.—(1) The fees payable under the Act are set out in the Schedule.

(2) Except for the initial annual membership fee, the annual membership fee is due on the 30th day of November in each year, for the following year.

(3) An educational licence is valid for six months and the fee for a renewal of an educational licence is due before the licence expires.

(4) The inspection fee payable in respect of a certificate of accreditation is due thirty days after the inspection is performed. R.R.O. 1990, Reg. 1093, s. 16.

PART II
PRACTICE STANDARDS

17.—(1) For the purposes of the Act, professional misconduct includes the following:

1. An act or omission inconsistent with the Act or this Regulation.

2. Failing to maintain the standard of practice of the profession.

3. Failing to fulfil the terms of an agreement with a client.

4. Failing to continue to provide professional services to an animal until the services are no longer required or until the client has had a reasonable opportunity to arrange for the services of another member.

5. Failing to provide within a reasonable time and without cause any certificate or report requested by a client or his or her agent in respect to an examination or treatment performed by the member.

6. Revealing information concerning an animal, or any professional service performed for an animal, to any person other than the client or another member except,

    i. with the consent of the client,

    ii. when required to do so by law, or

    iii. to prevent, or contribute information for the treatment of, a disease or physical injury of a person.

7. Providing, or attempting or offering to provide, services that are not reasonably useful or needed.

8. Making a misrepresentation to a client or prospective client.

9. Making a claim respecting the utility of any remedy, treatment, device or procedure other than a claim which can reasonably be supported as professional opinion.

10. Guaranteeing a cure, or making a statement which a client would reasonably understand as a guarantee of a cure.

11. Charging a fee that is excessive in relation to the services performed.

12. Charging a fee for an unperformed service, except a fee for an appointment missed without at least twenty-four hours notice.

13. Charging a fee for prescribing, but a member may charge a fee for advice to the client.

14. Adding a charge to a disbursement, but a member may charge a fee for the interpretation of the results of a laboratory investigation.

15. Knowingly submitting a false or misleading account or charge for professional services.

16. Failing to issue a statement or receipt when a statement or receipt is requested by a client or his or her agent.

17. Failing to itemize the services provided, the fees therefor and the disbursements charged, when an itemized account is requested by a client or his or her agent.

18. Reducing, or offering to reduce, an account for prompt payment without notifying the client of the terms of reduction before providing the pertinent service.

19. Charging interest on an account without notifying the client of the terms of interest before providing the pertinent service, except where interest has been granted by a court.

20. Selling, or attempting to sell, an account for professional services to a third party, but a member may retain a lawyer or agent to collect unpaid accounts and may accept payment for professional services by a credit card.

21. Failing to dispose of an animal, deceased or alive, or a part thereof, in accordance with the client's instructions if those instructions are in accordance with law and accepted veterinary standards and practice.

22. If a client fails to give instructions regarding disposal of an animal or a part thereof, or gives instructions not in accordance with law or accepted veterinary standards and practices, disposing of the animal or a part thereof by any means that are not in accordance with law and accepted veterinary standards and practices.

23. If an animal has died unexpectedly or from an anaesthetic, failing to promptly inform the client about the availability of a necropsy through a veterinarian independent of the attending veterinarian but, having provided the information, the attending veterinarian or an associate, upon the client's request, may perform the necropsy.

24. Abusing a client verbally or physically or permitting or counselling an associate or auxiliary to abuse a client verbally or physically.

25. Having a conflict of interest.

26. Having a licence under the *Livestock Medicines Act* or an interest in an establishment or undertaking that has a licence under that Act, or deriving a benefit directly or indirectly from an establishment or undertaking that has a licence under the *Livestock Medicines Act*.

27. Failing to make or retain the records required by this Regulation.

28. Falsifying a record regarding professional services.

29. Failing to abide by a condition in a licence or a certificate of accreditation.

30. Failing to direct or supervise, or inadequately directing or supervising, an auxiliary.

31. Permitting, counselling or assisting any person, other than a member, to practise, or to attempt to practise, veterinary medicine.

32. Permitting, advising or assisting any person, other than a member, to perform any act or function which should properly be performed by a member.

33. Directly or by implication representing any person to be a member who is not a member.

34. Signing or issuing a veterinary certificate, report or similar document that contains a statement that the member knows or ought to know is false, misleading or otherwise improper.

35. Signing or issuing a veterinary certificate, report or similar document without ascertaining, or taking reasonable measures to determine, the accuracy of its contents.

36. Permitting a veterinary certificate, report or similar document to be issued in the member's name, or with his or her concurrence, without personally signing it.

37. If a licence of another person is suspended or has been revoked or cancelled, a member for any purpose related to the practice of veterinary medicine, except with the prior written consent of the Executive Committee and subject to the terms of that consent,

    i. retains or uses the services of that person,

    ii. employs or is employed by him or her,

    iii. maintains a partnership or association with him or her,

    iv. directly or indirectly receives, makes or confers any remuneration or benefit from or to him or her, or

    v. shares or occupies space with him or her.

38. Failing to reply appropriately or within a reasonable time to a written inquiry received from the College.

39. Making any statement, orally or in writing, calculated to belittle or injure the professional reputation of another veterinarian, or unnecessarily commenting adversely upon any professional act of another veterinarian.

40. Treating an animal receiving veterinary services from another member without notifying the other member and obtaining the relevant historical information as soon as practicable.

41. Treating an animal receiving veterinary services from another member who did not refer the animal without advising the client that such uncoordinated veterinary services may place the animal at risk.

42. Engaging in or permitting the publication, broadcast, display, distribution or use of, a testimonial or endorsement.

43. Touting or, except as permitted by this Regulation, soliciting professional business.

44. An act or omission relevant to the practice of veterinary medicine that, having regard to the circumstances, would reasonably be regarded as unprofessional conduct.

(2) Despite paragraph 26 of subsection (1), it is not professional misconduct for a member to own shares in the United Co-Operatives of Ontario or in a corporation the shares of which are publicly traded through the Toronto Stock Exchange even if the corporation has a licence under the *Livestock Medicines Act*. R.R.O. 1990, Reg. 1093, s. 17.

18. A member shall exercise generally accepted standards of practice and procedures in the performance of veterinary services. R.R.O. 1990, Reg. 1093, s. 18.

19.—(1) A member is responsible for the conduct of his or her auxiliaries and for the suitability and quality of the performance of their acts.

(2) A member is guilty of professional misconduct if an auxiliary of the member does or omits to do anything that, if done or omitted by a member, would constitute professional misconduct.

(3) A member properly supervises the performance of an auxiliary's task if the member,

(a) is physically present on the premises when the task is performed, remains available for personal intervention if required and monitors the performance to determine that the task is properly carried out; or

(b) if absent on account of an emergency or otherwise temporarily absent and the performance of the task does not require a member's attendance, has given general instructions for such an occasion and the member ascertains as soon as practicable after the task is performed that it was properly carried out.

(4) A member may direct an auxiliary who is suitably qualified by education or experience to perform, under the supervision of a member, the tasks traditionally assigned to auxiliaries including flushing and infusion procedures in the course of embryo transfers after appropriate assessment by a member. R.R.O. 1990, Reg. 1093, s. 19.

20.—(1) A member is responsible for providing reasonably prompt services outside of regular practice hours if the services are medically necessary for animals that he or she has recently treated or that he or she treats regularly.

(2) The services required under subsection (1) may be provided by the member or an associate or by referral to another member who has agreed to cover the referring member's practice.

(3) If a member provides services under subsection (1) outside of regular practice hours by referring an animal to an emergency clinic, the member is responsible for promptly continuing to provide medically necessary services to the animal after discharge from the emergency clinic until the services are no longer required or until the client has had a reasonable opportunity to arrange for the services of another member. R.R.O. 1990, Reg. 1093, s. 20.

21.—(1) A member who induces general anaesthesia in an animal or undertakes critical care of an animal is responsible for monitoring the recovery of the animal until its medical condition is stable and satisfactory.

(2) The monitoring under subsection (1) may be done personally, through another member or through an auxiliary who is suitably qualified by education or experience if supervised by the member. R.R.O. 1990, Reg. 1093, s. 21.

22.—(1) The records required in respect of each companion animal shall contain the following information:

1. Patient identification, including species, age and sex.

2. The client's name, address and telephone numbers.

3. If the client is likely to be absent from his or her address while the animal is confined with the member, the name, address and telephone number of a person to be contacted in case of an emergency.

4. Date of each time that the member sees the animal.

5. A history of the animal's health, including a record of vaccinations.

6. The animal's current weight.

7. Particulars of each assessment, including any laboratory investigations, performed or ordered by the member and the results of each assessment.

8. A note of any professional advice given regarding the animal and an indication of when and to whom such advice was given if other than to the client.

9. All medical or surgical treatments and procedures used, dispensed, prescribed or performed by or at the direction of the member, including the name, strength, dose and quantity of any drugs.

10. A copy of all reports prepared by the member in respect of the animal.

11. A final assessment of the animal.

12. The fees and charges, showing separately those for drugs and those for advice or other services.

13. Any additional records required by this Regulation.

(2) The records required in respect of each food-producing animal or herd shall contain the following information:

1. Individual or herd identification, or both, including species, breed and sex.

2. If individual advice or care is given, at least one of the animal's name, the animal's tattoo or ear-tag number or the animal's colour, markings or other distinguishing physical features.

3. The client's name, address and telephone numbers.

4. The name and telephone number of a person to be contacted in the absence of the client.

5. Date of each service.

6. A history of the presenting complaint.

7. If there is a presenting complaint, particulars of each assessment, including any laboratory investigations performed or ordered by the member and the results of each assessment.

8. A note of any professional advice regarding the individual or herd and an indication of to whom the advice was given if other than to the client.

9. A complete record of all written prescriptions and drugs dispensed or prescribed by the member in accordance with section 26.

10. A copy of any report prepared by the member in respect of the individual or herd.

11. The fees and charges, showing separately those for drugs and those for advice or other services.

12. Any additional records required by this Regulation.

(3) The records required in respect of a horse are the same as those required in respect of a food-producing animal.

(4) The records required in respect of poultry, for each bird or flock, shall contain the following information:

1. Bird or flock identification, or both, including species and type.

2. The client's name, address and telephone numbers.

3. The name and telephone number of a person to be contacted in the absence of the client.

4. Date of each service.

5. A history of the presenting complaint.

6. If there is a presenting complaint, particulars of each assessment, including any laboratory investigations performed or ordered by the member and the results of each assessment.

7. A note of any professional advice regarding the bird or flock and an indication of to whom the advice was given if other than to the client.

8. A complete record of all written prescriptions and drugs dispensed or prescribed by the member, made in accordance with section 27.

9. A copy of any report prepared by the member in respect of the bird or flock.

10. The fees and charges showing separately those for drugs and those for advice or other services.

11. Any additional records required by this Regulation.

(5) The records required under this section shall be,

(a) legibly written or typewritten;

(b) kept in a systematic manner; and

(c) retained for a period of at least five years after the date of the last entry in the record or until two years after the member ceases to practise veterinary medicine, whichever occurs first.

(6) Despite subsection (5), the records required under this section may be maintained in any electronic medium that provides a visual display of recorded information if,

(a) the recorded information is capable of being printed promptly; and

(b) any changes in the recorded information are clearly indicated as changes. R.R.O. 1990, Reg. 1093, s. 22.

PART III
DRUGS

23.—(1) In this Part,

''controlled drug'' means any drug or substance included in Schedule G;

''dispense'' means administer, sell, distribute or give away;

''drug'' means a drug as defined in subsection 117 (1) of the *Health Disciplines Act*;

''internal use'' means local or systemic absorption upon introduction into the body by the parenteral route or through a body orifice;

''narcotic'' means any substance included in Schedule N or anything that contains a substance included in Schedule N;

''pharmacist'' means a person who is licensed under Part IV of the *Health Disciplines Act*;

''prescription'' means the dispensing of any drug or mixture of drugs.

(2) A reference to Schedule B, D, E, F, G or N is a reference to such Schedule established by Regulation 551 of Revised Regulations of Ontario, 1990 made under Part VI of the *Health Disciplines Act*. R.R.O. 1990, Reg. 1093, s. 23.

24. Subsections 22 (5) and (6) apply to the registers, entries and other records required by this Part. R.R.O. 1990, Reg. 1093, s. 24.

25.—(1) Every member who dispenses drugs shall maintain a system for filing the records of the purchase and dispensing of the drugs.

(2) A member shall keep a record of every purchase of a drug and, immediately upon such purchase shall enter,

(a) the date of the purchase;

(b) the name, strength and quantity of the drug;

(c) the name and address of the person from whom the drug was purchased or received;

(d) the purchase price; and

(e) in the case of a controlled drug or narcotic, the signature of the member who made the purchase.

(3) The maintenance in systematic order of all drug purchase invoices is a record for the purposes of subsection (2). R.R.O. 1990, Reg. 1093, s. 25.

26. If a member decides to treat an animal with a drug and either does not dispense it or is asked by the owner for a prescription, the member shall give a written prescription to the owner or offer to give an oral prescription to a pharmacist acceptable to the owner. R.R.O. 1990, Reg. 1093, s. 26.

27.—(1) A member who dispenses a drug shall make a written record showing,

(a) the name and address of the owner of the animal or group of animals for which the drug is prescribed;

(b) the name, strength and quantity of the prescribed drug;

(c) the directions for use if they are different than the directions for use on the manufacturer's label or if the manufacturer's label does not specify the directions for use;

(d) the date on which the drug is dispensed; and

(e) the price charged.

(2) The member shall retain the written record required under subsection (1) for a period of at least five years or until he or she ceases to practice veterinary medicine, whichever occurs first.

(3) A member who dispenses a drug shall mark the container in which the drug is dispensed with,

(a) the name, strength and quantity of the drug;

(b) the date the drug is dispensed;

(c) the name and address of the member;

(d) the identity of the animal or group of animals for which it is dispensed;

(e) the name of the owner of the animal or animals; and

(f) the prescribed directions for use.

(4) Except for a drug referred to in Schedule G or N or Part I of Schedule F, subsection (3) does not apply if the container in which a drug is dispensed is the original and unopened container in which the drug was packaged, the original label on the container has not been altered and the prescribed directions for use are the same as the directions for use on the original label. R.R.O. 1990, Reg. 1093, s. 27.

28.—(1) A member who dispenses a drug referred to in Schedule G or N shall keep a narcotics and controlled drug register in which is entered,

(a) the date of the dispensing;

(b) the name and address of the owner of the animal or animals for which the drug was dispensed;

(c) the name, strength and quantity of the drug dispensed;

(d) the quantity of the drug remaining after dispensing; and

(e) the price charged.

(2) A member shall,

(a) protect controlled drugs and narcotics in his or her possession from loss and theft;

(b) report immediately any loss or theft of a controlled drug or narcotic to a police officer; and

(c) report any loss or theft of a controlled drug or narcotic within ten days of the discovery thereof to the Minister of Health and Welfare, Canada.

(3) A member shall not permit any person other than another member or an auxiliary acting upon the specific direction of a member to dispense or have access to a controlled drug or narcotic.

(4) Controlled drugs and narcotics shall be kept in a locked cabinet designed and constructed to ensure the reasonable security of the drugs.

(5) The cabinet mentioned in subsection (4) shall be kept locked except when drugs are being placed in or removed from the cabinet.

(6) A member shall not prescribe or dispense a controlled drug or narcotic unless,

(a) the animal for which the controlled drug or narcotic is prescribed or dispensed is an animal under his or her professional treatment; and

(b) the controlled drug or narcotic is required for a condition for which the animal is receiving treatment from the member. R.R.O. 1990, Reg. 1093, s. 28.

29.—(1) A member who dispenses a drug referred to in Part I of Schedule D shall keep a poison register in which is entered,

(a) the date of the dispensing;

(b) the name and address of the purchaser;

(c) the name, strength and quantity of the drug dispensed; and

(d) the purpose for which the drug is required as stated by the purchaser.

(2) No drug referred to in Part I of Schedule D shall be delivered to the purchaser until the record required under subsection (1) has been completed and both the purchaser and member have signed the record.

(3) A member who dispenses a drug referred to in Part I of Schedule D shall ensure that the name of the drug and the word "POISON" is legibly and conspicuously displayed on the outer surface of the container of the drug.

(4) A member who dispenses a drug referred to in Part II of Schedule D for internal use shall ensure that the name of the drug and the words "*CAUTION: May be poisonous if used in large doses or for a long time. Do not exceed the recommended dose without consulting a veterinarian*" are legibly and conspicuously displayed on the outer surface of the container of the drug.

(5) A member who dispenses a drug referred to in Part II of Schedule D for external application shall ensure that the name of the drug and the words "*CAUTION: FOR EXTERNAL APPLICATION ONLY: May be poisonous if used internally*" are legibly and conspicuously displayed on the outer surface of the container of the drug. R.R.O. 1990, Reg. 1093, s. 29.

30.—(1) A member shall not dispense a substance listed in Schedule B unless it is labelled in accordance with this section.

(2) A container in which a substance referred to in Part II of Schedule B is dispensed shall include on the label, legibly and conspicuously displayed on the outer surface of the container, the name of the substance and a caution or warning that the substance should be kept out of reach of children.

(3) A container in which a substance referred to in Part III of Schedule B is dispensed shall include on the label, legibly and conspicuously displayed on the outer surface of the container, the name of the substance and a caution or warning that the substance should be used only with adequate ventilation.

(4) Subsections (2) and (3) do not apply if the substance is referred to in the *Hazardous Products Act* (Canada). R.R.O. 1990, Reg. 1093, s. 30.

31.—(1) In this section, "withholding time" means, in reference to an animal that receives a drug or substance, the period of time for which the animal or the product of the animal should be withheld or withdrawn from sale for consumption.

(2) When a member dispenses a drug or substance for use in food-producing animals, the member shall advise the recipient of the drug or substance of an appropriate withholding time, which shall be at least as long as the withholding time recommended by the manufacturer of the drug or substance.

(3) The container in which the drug or substance is dispensed shall include on the label, legibly and conspicuously displayed on the outer surface of the container, a warning of an appropriate withholding time, which shall be at least as long as the withholding time recommended by the manufacturer.

(4) When a member dispenses a drug or substance for use in food-producing animals and the member knows or suspects that use will be made or a dosage will be administered of the drug or substance that is different than the use or dosage that is customary or recommended by the manufacturer, the member shall, in addition to the advice required under subsection (2), advise the recipient of the drug or substance that the appropriate withholding time is not known but should be substantially longer than the recommended withholding time. R.R.O. 1990, Reg. 1093, s. 31.

32.—(1) In this section, "child resistant package" means a container or package that meets the requirements of the regulations made under the *Food and Drugs Act* (Canada).

(2) A member shall dispense a drug in a child resistant package unless,

(a) a child resistant package is unobtainable through no fault of the member; or

(b) a child resistant package is not suitable because of the amount or physical form of the drug. R.R.O. 1990, Reg. 1093, s. 32.

33.—(1) No member shall administer, dispense or prescribe a drug unless,

(a) the member has assumed the responsibility for making medical judgements regarding the health of the animal and the need for medical treatment and the custodian of the animal has indicated a willingness to accept the advice of the member;

(b) the member has sufficient knowledge of the animal by virtue of a history and inquiry and either physical examination of the animal or medically appropriate and timely visits to the premises where the animal is kept to reach at least a general or preliminary diagnosis;

(c) the member believes that the drug is prophylactically or thera-peutically indicated for the animal; and

(d) the member is readily available in case of adverse reactions to the drug or failure of the regimen of therapy. R.R.O. 1990, Reg. 1093, s. 33 (1).

(2) No member shall,

(a) sign a blank prescription form;

(b) knowingly represent that a drug is a drug which it is not or that it contains a substance which it does not;

(c) send through the mail, except by registered mail, a drug referred to in Schedule D, E, F, G or N;

(d) knowingly dispense a drug for resale except to another member or a pharmacist;

(e) dispense a drug or possess a drug for the purpose of dispensing the drug at any place other than a veterinary facility where he or she regularly practises veterinary medicine; or

(f) dispense Hoechst Pharmaceutical product T-61 except for administration by a member or by a person known by the member to be competent at intravenous injection,

(i) who is an auxiliary of the member acting upon the specific direction of the member, or

(ii) who is carrying out euthanasia duties while operating, or while being employed by a person operating a pound or research facility, within the meaning of the *Animals for Research Act*. R.R.O. 1990, Reg. 1093, s. 33 (2); O. Reg. 407/92, s. 5.

PART IV
HOLDING OUT

34. In this Part, "ancillary services" means boarding, grooming, funeral services and sales of foods, supplies and other goods and services used by or with animals that is provided by a member whether as part of, or separately from, his or her practice of veterinary medicine. R.R.O. 1990, Reg. 1093, s. 34.

35. No member shall publish, display, distribute or use, or permit, directly or indirectly, the publication, display, distribution or use of any advertisement, announcement or similar form of communication related to the member's professional services or ancillary services or to a member's association with, or employment by, any person, except as permitted by this Part. R.R.O. 1990, Reg. 1093, s. 35.

36.—(1) Except as provided in this Part, a member may communicate factual, accurate and verifiable information that a reasonable person would consider relevant in the choice of a veterinarian, including the availability of ancillary services, that,

(a) is not false, misleading or deceptive by the inclusion or omission of any information;

(b) is readily comprehensible, dignified and in good taste;

(c) contains no testimonial or comparative statements;

(d) contains no information in respect of a fee or price; and

(e) contains no reference to a specific drug, appliance or equipment.

(2) Despite clause (1) (d), a member may display or distribute within the veterinary facility where he or she practises a fee schedule stating the fee for some or all professional services or ancillary services or an explanation of the basis for the calculation of such fees, or both.

(3) The location and size of a displayed fee schedule permitted by subsection (2) shall be such that it cannot be read by a person outside the veterinary facility. R.R.O. 1990, Reg. 1093, s. 36.

(4) No information shall be communicated using a medium that is not equally accessible to all interested members to use.   O. Reg. 308/91, s. 2.

37.—(1) A member shall not cause or permit, directly or indirectly, his or her name to appear in any communication offering to the public any product or service other than the member's professional services and ancillary services.

(2) A member shall not be associated with the advertising or promotion of any product or service other than the member's professional services and ancillary services.

(3) Despite subsections (1) and (2), a member may be associated with the advertising of a product or service and permit his or her name to appear in a communication offering to the public a product or service in a printed publication intended to be read principally by veterinarians. R.R.O. 1990, Reg. 1093, s. 37.

38.   A member shall not participate directly or indirectly in a system in which another person steers or recommends clients to a member for a professional service or an ancillary service.   R.R.O. 1990, Reg. 1093, s. 38.

39.   A member shall not contact or communicate with, or attempt to contact or communicate with, any person in order to solicit patronage of professional services or ancillary services.   R.R.O. 1990, Reg. 1093, s. 39.

40.—(1) Despite section 39, a member may,

(a) send written communications, consistent with subsection 36 (1), generally to persons not known to need professional services or ancillary services but who might in general find the availability of such services useful;

(b) distribute to his or her regular clients general information about animal health, preventive medicine and recent developments in veterinary medicine; and

(c) inform his or her regular clients, in writing or by telephone, about health maintenance procedures that are due to be carried out, including a due date for immunization.   R.R.O. 1990, Reg. 1093, s. 40 (1); O. Reg. 308/91, s. 3.

(2) For the purposes of subsection (1),

(a) a person is a regular client of a member if,

(i) the person uses the professional services of the member regularly and with reasonable frequency, and

(ii) the person has not requested the transfer of the records for the person's animal to another member; and

(b) a person who uses the professional services of a member who is in the employment of another member shall be deemed to be a client only of the employer member.

(3) A communication authorized by clause (1) (a) shall be clearly and prominently marked "advertisement" on each page.   R.R.O. 1990, Reg. 1093, s. 40 (2, 3).

41.—(1) The name used by a member in the practice of veterinary medicine shall be the same as the name in which the member is entered in the register.

(2) A member may name the veterinary facility in which he or she carries on an independent or private practice of veterinary medicine with a designation approved by the Accreditation Committee.

(3) The designation under subsection (2) shall contain,

(a) a geographical reference appropriate to the location of the facility or the surname of a member who is or was associated with the practice;

(b) the word "animal", "pet" or "veterinary" except,

(i) if the practice in or from the facility is restricted to one particular species, the name of that species or one of the words "animal", "pet" or "veterinary" or both the name of the species and one of the words "animal", "pet" and "veterinary", and

(ii) if the practice in or from the facility is restricted to poultry, the word "poultry" with or without the word "veterinary"; and

(c) an appropriate term required under section 11 for the class of certificate of accreditation of the facility.

(4) The Accreditation Committee shall not approve the designation if it is of the opinion that the proposed designation,

(a) is inconsistent with subsection (3);

(b) is improper or unfitting; or

(c) may tend to be confused with the designation of another veterinary facility.

(5) The approval of the Accreditation Committee is not required in respect of a designation that conforms to subsection (3) and that was in use on the 16th day of November, 1985.   R.R.O. 1990, Reg. 1093, s. 41.

PART V
CONFLICT OF INTEREST

42.—(1) In this Part, "related person" means a person connected with a member by blood relationship, marriage or adoption, and,

(a) persons are connected by blood relationship if one is the child or other descendent of the other or one is the brother or sister of the other;

(b) persons are connected by marriage if one is married to the other or to a person who is connected by blood relationship to the other; and

(c) persons are connected by adoption if one has been adopted, either legally or in fact, as the child of the other or as the child of a person who is so connected by blood relationship, except as a brother or sister, to the other.

(2) A member has a conflict of interest where the member, or a related person, or an employee or employer of the member, directly or indirectly,

(a) enters into any agreement, including a lease of premises, under which any amount payable by or to a member or a related person is related to the amount of fees charged by the member; or

(b) receives, makes or confers a fee, credit or other benefit by reason of the referral or transfer of an animal or a specimen from or to any other person.

(3) Despite clause (2) (a), a member may enter into a partnership agreement with another member under which the drawings, interest or remuneration of the partners is related to the amount of fees charged by them.   R.R.O. 1990, Reg. 1093, s. 42.

43.—(1) In this section,

"employee" includes an agent;

"employer" includes a principal.

(2) A member has a conflict of interest who performs a veterinary service in the course of employment by any person, other than another member, except a service provided to the member's employer or in accordance with subsection (4).

(3) For the purposes of subsection (2),

(a) a member who performs a veterinary service for an animal shall be deemed to perform the service to the owner of the animal which received the service; and

(b) a member employed by a humane society operated in accordance with the *Ontario Society for the Prevention of Cruelty to Animals Act* or by a pound operated under the *Animals for Research Act* who performs a veterinary service for an animal seized by, or irrevocably surrendered to, the society or pound shall be deemed to perform the service to his or her employer.

(4) A member may practise veterinary medicine as,

(a) an employee of the Crown in right of Canada or of Ontario or an agency of the Crown;

(b) an employee of the Ontario Veterinary College of the University of Guelph;

(c) an employee of a municipal corporation if, in the course of such employment, the member's practice with respect to animals not owned by the corporation is limited to spay and neuter procedures, including the pre-operative, intra-operative and post-operative management usually associated with such procedures;

(d) an employee of an individual, partnership or corporation selling food or drug products for use in food-producing animals if, in the course of the employment,

    (i) the member performs professional services related only to the employer's products and only for an established customer of the employer and at the customer's farm or similar establishment, and

    (ii) the member takes all reasonable steps to notify the normally attending veterinarian of the member's proposed visit and the reasons for it so that the normally attending veterinarian can discuss the matter with his or her client, and, if desirable, arrange to meet the member before or at the visit;

(e) an employee of a humane society operated in accordance with the *Ontario Society for the Prevention of Cruelty to Animals Act* if, in the course of the employment, the member provides professional services under a written contract that provides that the member is responsible for all decisions relating to the quality and promotion of the member's professional services and the health of the subject animals;

(f) an employee of Eastern Breeders Inc., United Breeders Inc. or Western Ontario Breeders Inc., while it holds a licence under the *Artificial Insemination of Livestock Act*, if, in the course of the employment, the member's practice with respect to animals not owned by the corporation is limited to services in respect of fertility, including ova and embryo transfer; and

(g) an employee of the personal representative of a deceased member or the guardian of an impaired member for a reasonable period of time after the member's death or the commencement of the member's impairment to settle matters. R.R.O. 1990, Reg. 1093, s. 43.

44.—(1) A member has a conflict of interest if the member or a partner or associate of the member,

(a) inspects or assesses an animal on behalf of both the seller and the buyer of the animal; or

(b) being regularly engaged by the seller or buyer of an animal, inspects or assesses an animal on behalf of the other party to a sale.

(2) Despite subsection (1), a member, or a partner or associate of the member, may inspect or assess an animal on behalf of both the buyer and seller of the animal or, where one or more of them are regularly engaged by the seller or buyer of an animal, any of them may inspect or assess an animal on behalf of the other party to a sale if, before accepting engagement by the second party, he or she,

(a) informs both parties of the conflict of interest and of the circumstances giving rise to it;

(b) informs both parties that no information received by the member, or a partner or associate of the member, in connection with the transaction can be treated as confidential so far as the other party is concerned; and

(c) after informing the parties under clauses (a) and (b), obtains the consent of both parties to inspect or assess the animal on behalf of both of them, which shall be in writing unless it is impracticable to obtain the consent in written form. R.R.O. 1990, Reg. 1093, s. 44.

PART VI
EXEMPTIONS

45.—(1) If a member or group of members sponsors a program to vaccinate domestic animals in order to reduce human exposure to rabies, the member may advertise the location, date and time of the program, the names of participating members and the cost of the vaccination if,

(a) all members practising in the area are invited to participate in the program at least two weeks before the vaccinations are to be carried out;

(b) the co-operation of the medical officer or officers of health for the area is requested; and

(c) the Registrar is given written notification of the program at least two weeks before the vaccinations are to be carried out and the notice confirms that there has been compliance with clauses (a) and (b).

(2) The vaccinations carried out in a program under subsection (1) need not be performed in an accredited veterinary facility if,

(a) drugs suitable for use in conventional veterinary emergencies are available on the premises where the program is being conducted;

(b) vaccines are kept refrigerated;

(c) the premises where the program is being conducted are kept clean; and

(d) vaccines are administered by an aseptic technique.

(3) The records in section 22 are not required in respect of a vaccination carried out in a program under subsection (1), but a member shall record,

(a) a reasonable identification of the vaccinated animal;

(b) the owner's name, address and telephone numbers;

(c) the date and fact of vaccination; and

(d) the type of vaccine, including the lot and serial number of the vaccine administered.

(4) The information recorded under subsection (3) shall be maintained in a systematic manner by the members organizing the program.

(5) A conventional assessment is not required before a vaccination is performed under this Part.

(6) After the vaccination, the member shall sign and give to the custodian of each vaccinated animal a certificate of vaccination for that animal, which shall legibly set out the name and telephone number of the vaccinating member. R.R.O. 1990, Reg. 1093, s. 45.

PART VII
ADMINISTRATION

46. Every member, other than a member who holds a short term licence, shall submit to the College by the 30th day of November in each year, an information return setting out,

(a) the member's principal place of practice or principal place of residence;

(b) the address to which the member wishes correspondence from the College to be sent;

(c) the addresses and telephone numbers of all locations where the member practises veterinary medicine;

(d) the nature of the member's veterinary practice during the twelve-month period ending on the 31st day of October; and

(e) the professional associates of the member and the form of relationship between them and the member. R.R.O. 1990, Reg. 1093, s. 46.

47.—(1) Before the 31st day of October in each year, the Registrar shall mail to each member, other than a member who holds a short term or educational licence, a notice stating that the annual membership fee and a completed annual information return are due on the 30th day of November and setting out the amount of the fee.

(2) The Registrar shall mail to each member who holds an educational licence,

(a) at least one month before the licence is due to expire, a notice setting out the due date and amount of the renewal fee; and

(b) before the 31st day of October in each year, a notice stating that a completed annual information return is due on the 30th day of November.

(3) The obligation to pay the annual membership fee or renewal fee and to submit the annual information return continues even if the Registrar fails to mail a notice under subsection (1) or (2) or the member fails to receive such notice. R.R.O. 1990, Reg. 1093, s. 47.

48.—(1) A member in private practice in Ontario shall maintain a principal place of practice.

(2) A member shall notify the Registrar in writing of the address to which the member wishes correspondence from the college to be sent and shall notify the Registrar in writing of any change of address.

(3) A member who is in private practice in Ontario shall notify the Registrar in writing of the municipal address or lot and concession number of his or her principal place of practice and shall notify the Registrar in writing of any change in such place.

(4) A member who is not in private practice in Ontario shall notify the Registrar in writing of the municipal address, lot and concession number or other physical location of his or her principal place of practice or principal place of residence and shall notify the Registrar in writing of every change in such place.

(5) If a member fails to comply with this section, the address to which the member wishes correspondence from the College to be sent and the member's principal place of practice or residence shall be deemed to be as shown on the last information return submitted under section 46. R.R.O. 1990, Reg. 1093, s. 48.

49.—(1) The Executive Committee shall regularly determine what statistical information is desirable on the supply, distribution and professional activities of members of the College and may direct the Registrar to compile the desired information.

(2) Upon the written request of the Registrar, a member shall provide to the Registrar the information requested for the compilation of statistics. R.R.O. 1990, Reg. 1093, s. 49.

50.—(1) The Registrar shall cause, and the members shall permit, the inspection of facilities and of the records kept by members in connection with the practice of veterinary medicine, in order to determine if,

(a) the facility is being operated under and in accordance with a certificate of accreditation;

(b) the facility and the applicant or holder of a certificate of accreditation meet the qualifications and requirements for a certificate of accreditation;

(c) the records in respect of the practice of veterinary medicine are being kept as required; and

(d) the veterinary medicine being practised is generally in accordance with the standards of practice of the profession.

(2) A holder of a certificate of accreditation who meets the requirements of section 10 is eligible for a renewal of the certificate if an application for the renewal is submitted not earlier than five months and not later than three months before the expiry of the certificate.

(3) If an application for renewal is not submitted in the time specified under subsection (2) and the certificate of accreditation expires, the holder of the certificate must submit a new application.

(4) Upon receipt of an application for renewal, the Registrar shall promptly cause an inspection under subsection (1) to be carried out.

(5) If a holder of a certificate of accreditation applies in accordance with subsection (2), and the inspection does not occur one month or more before the expiry of the certificate of accreditation, the certificate of accreditation remains valid,

(a) until the Registrar renews the certificate of accreditation; or

(b) where the Registrar refuses to renew the certificate of accreditation, until the Accreditation Committee decides the disposition of the application.

(6) If a member applies for a certificate of accreditation and complies with clauses 10 (a) to (d), the Registrar shall promptly cause an inspection to be carried out in order to determine if the veterinary facility meets the applicable standards established under subsection 8 (1) of the Act. R.R.O. 1990, Reg. 1093, s. 50.

51.—(1) Subject to subsection (2), the name of a member entered in the register shall be the same as the name of the member in the documentary evidence of his or her basic degree in veterinary medicine.

(2) The Registrar shall direct the entry of a name other than the name required by subsection (1) if the member satisfies the Registrar that the use of the other name is not for an improper purpose and deposits with the College,

(a) a certified copy of an order of a court of competent jurisdiction in Ontario changing the member's name or a change of name certificate issued under the *Change of Name Act*;

(b) a certified copy of a valid certificate of marriage or of a decree absolute of divorce from a court in Canada;

(c) documentary material that, in the opinion of the Registrar, sufficiently identifies the member as the person named in the documentary evidence of his or her basic degree in veterinary medicine; or

(d) any combination of material referred to in clauses (a), (b) and (c).

(3) Subsection (2) applies with necessary modifications to an applicant for a licence. R.R.O. 1990, Reg. 1093, s. 51.

52. The Registrar shall enter in the register the principal place of practice or residence of each member. R.R.O. 1990, Reg. 1093, s. 52.

53.—(1) Any person may inspect the information entered in the register or in the directory during the normal hours of operation of the College's offices.

(2) The register or the directory may be maintained in an electronic form and, if so, the information entered in the register or in the directory shall be capable of being printed promptly.

(3) The Registrar may give information from the register or the directory to any person in printed form or orally. R.R.O. 1990, Reg. 1093, s. 53.

54.—(1) The Registrar shall issue a certificate of standing in respect of a member to any person who requests a certificate and pays the appropriate fee set out in the Schedule.

(2) A certificate of standing shall set out,

(a) the information respecting the member that is entered in the register; and

(b) whether there is any outstanding referral to the Discipline Committee or the Registration Committee in respect of the member. R.R.O. 1990, Reg. 1093, s. 54.

55.—(1) The Registrar shall publish the written reasons for any decision of the Discipline Committee in the original or a modified form and, in any such publication,

(a) the identity of the member shall be made known if the name of the member or former member is required by the Act to be included in the publication of the Committee's finding; or

(b) if clause (a) does not apply, the identity of the member shall not be made known unless the member requests in writing that he or she be identified.

(2) The written reasons for a decision of the Discipline Committee, in their original or modified form, shall be available to the public upon request.

(3) The Registrar may communicate orally or in writing, or both, the decision of the Discipline Committee to any complainant and upon request, to any witness who testified at the hearing and the Registrar may also provide any other information necessary to explain the proceedings and the decision to the complainant or witness, including a copy of any written reasons of the committee in their original or modified form.

(4) The Registrar may publish the findings and reasons for a decision of the Registration Committee in respect of impairment proceedings but, in any such publication, the identity of any member who is the subject of impairment proceedings shall not be made known. R.R.O. 1990, Reg. 1093, s. 55.

Schedule

FEES

1.	Local examination	$100.00
2.	Application fee:	
	(a) for short term or educational licence	25.00
	(b) for all other licences	50.00
3.	Licence fee:	
	(a) for short term or educational licence	nil
	(b) for all other licences	50.00
4.	Membership fee:	
	(a) for short term licence	100.00
	(b) for educational licence for six months	50.00
	(c) for all other licences	525.00
5.	Initial annual membership fee where licence is issued:	
	(a) between April 1st and June 30th	300.00
	(b) between July 1st and September 30th	200.00
	(c) between October 1st and December 31st	100.00

6. Annual membership fee, excluding the intitial annual membership fee, for a member holding a general licence but who resides outside of Ontario and does not practice veterinary medicine in Ontario 200.00

7. Penalty for late payment of,

  (a) an annual membership fee 100.00

  (b) a fee for an educational licence 25.00

8. Inspection administrative fee 75.00

9. Inspection fees, in addition to the amount specified in Item 8:

  (a) for the inspection of a companion animal hospital, a companion animal emergency clinic, a food-producing animal hospital or an equine clinic. .   75.00

  (b) for the inspection of a companion animal office, companion animal mobile office, companion animal spay-neuter clinic or a poultry service . .   60.00

  (c) for the inspection of a companion animal mobile, a food-producing animal mobile, an equine mobile or an equine emergency mobile 50.00

  (d) for the inspection mentioned in clause (c) if another facility is being inspected at the same time for the purposes of being accredited 35.00

  (e) for an inspection of two or more mobiles under clause (c) of the same kind, at the same location and at the same time 50.00
for the first mobile; $35 for each additional mobile

10. Penalty for late payment of a fee for inspection of one location 75.00

11. Certificate of standing 10.00

R.R.O. 1990, Reg. 1093, Sched.; O. Reg. 407/92, s. 6.

APPENDIX H

Sample Termination Letter

FANTASY VETERINARY CLINIC
123 Main Street
Anyville, Ontario
L1L 8V9

(111) 123 - 4567

August 23, 1994

Without Prejudice

Ms. Jane White,
345 King Street,
Anyville, Ontario
L1L 2V8

Dear Jane:

Re.: Termination of Employment

Further to our office conference today this will confirm that your employment with Fantasy Veterinary Clinic has been terminated effective immediately. I regret that this action is necessary; however, as you know, the current recessionary environment has called upon our clinic to reduce its overhead so as to sustain the downturn in the economy.

The following represents my proposal to you relating to the termination of your employment:

Termination Payment

I am prepared to pay to you the sum of $6,400.00 gross salary representing four months salary in lieu of notice of termination. This payment would be subject to all usual statutory deductions and would be payable in accordance with the usual bi-weekly payment dates, the first such payment to commence on September 1, 1994. In the event that you obtain other employment while these payments are outstanding I will pay to you one-half of the amount outstanding as of the date you commence your new employment, such payment to be made in a lump sum. In the event that you do not obtain other employment, the payments will cease on December 23, 1994.

Employment Counselling

In addition to the termination payment referred to above I will also pay for you to obtain employment counselling up to a maximum of $1,000.00.

Benefits

You will be entitled to receive all benefits, except long term disability coverage, until the earlier of the date that you commence new employment or December 23, 1994.

Recommendation

To assist your job search, I will provide you with an unqualified letter of recommendation outlining your job functions and history with Fantasy Veterinary Clinic.

Release

In the event that the terms of this arrangement are satisfactory to you I will require that you sign a form of release absolving me from any further liability with respect to your termination. You should seek independent legal and accounting advice prior to signing the release.

Irrevocable Date

This proposal is open for acceptance by you until August 30, 1994 at 3:00 p.m. failing which this offer shall be deemed to have been withdrawn and of no further effect.

Jane, I regret that this action is necessary and hope that you find the terms of this correspondence acceptable to you.

Yours very truly,

FANTASY VETERINARY CLINIC

per. John Black, DVM

APPENDIX I

Employment Agreement (Professional)

THIS EMPLOYMENT AGREEMENT made this 5th day of February, 1994.

BETWEEN:

IMA NEWGUY
(herein referred to as the "Employee")

OF THE FIRST PART

- and -

JOHN WHITE and JANE BLACK
Carrying on business in partnership under the firm
name and style of "Fantasy Veterinary Services"
(herein referred to as the "Employer")

OF THE SECOND PART

WHEREAS the Employer is a professional partnership of John White and Jane Black who carry on the practice of veterinary medicine in partnership from its principal place of business being 123 Main Street, Anywhere Ontario;

AND WHEREAS the Employee has been granted his Doctor of Veterinary Medicine degree and is a member in good standing of the College of Veterinarians of Ontario;

AND WHEREAS the Employer has agreed to employ the Employee on the terms and conditions hereinafter set forth.

NOW THEREFORE THIS AGREEMENT WITNESSETH that in consideration of the covenants, agreements and promises herein set forth and other good and valuable consideration, the receipt and sufficiency of which is by the parties hereto acknowledged, THE PARTIES AGREE AS FOLLOWS:

1.00   EMPLOYMENT OF EMPLOYEE

1.01   Employment

The Employer agrees to employ the Employee and the Employee agrees to provide services to the Employer in accordance with the terms of this Agreement.

1.02   Agency

The Employee hereby acknowledges that he does not act as an agent nor does any agency relationship exist between himself and the Employer and agrees that he shall not represent himself to be the agent of the Employer for any purpose and shall not incur any obligation or make any promise or representation on behalf of the Employer. Further, the Employee agrees to indemnify and save harmless the Employer against any damages, suits, actions, or causes of actions directly or indirectly arising out of any representations the Employee makes that he acts as an agent for the Employer.

1.03   Obligations of Employee

Unless prevented by ill health or other sufficient cause, the Employee, during the Term (as hereinafter defined) and every renewal thereof, shall devote his full time and attention to the business of the Employer, and shall not, without written permission of the Employer, directly or indirectly, engage in any other business of any other corporation, firm or individual.

1.04 Confidentiality

(a) The Employee shall well and faithfully serve the Employer and use his best efforts to promote the interest thereof, and shall not disclose the private affairs of the Employer or any secret of the Employer to any person, other than the officers of the Employer, and shall not use for his own purpose, or for any purpose other than those of the Employer, any information he may acquire with respect to the Employer's affairs.

(b) All information, documents, customer data and like material are hereby deemed to be confidential.

1.05 Non-Competition

(a) Upon termination of the Employee's employment or of this Agreement the Employee agrees that, for a period of two (2) years following such termination, he shall not either directly or indirectly, alone or as a member of a partnership, engage in the practice of veterinary medicine, nor deal directly with any client of the Employer within the City of Anywhere and a twenty (20) kilometre radius thereof.

(b) The term "client" as employed in subparagraph (a) hereof shall be deemed to be any party for whom the Employer has rendered professional veterinary services within a period of two (2) years prior to the termination referred to in subparagraph (a).

(c) The Employee acknowledges and agrees that the restrictions contained in subparagraph (a) are reasonable in the circumstances and necessary for the protection of the integrity of the Employer and agrees that he shall not challenge this covenant in any subsequent court action based in law or equity and that this clause may be raised as an estoppel to any such challenge.

1.06 Automobile and Expenses

(a) The Employee shall provide his own automobile suitable to carry out the performance of the obligations of the Employee pursuant to this Agreement and shall be granted a car allowance of thirty-one cents ($0.31) per kilometre travelled plus parking expenses actually incurred by him in the performance of his duties (the "Automobile Expenses").

(b)   The Automobile Expenses shall be paid by the Employer to the Employee no later than the fifteenth (15th) day of the month subsequent to the month to which the Automobile Expenses relate.

1.07   Other Expenses

The Employee hereby acknowledges that, save and except any expenses otherwise provided for in this Agreement, he shall be solely responsible for the payment of any expenses incurred in connection with the services performed by him pursuant to this Agreement and that the Employer shall not be required to reimburse the Employee for any expenses so incurred.

1.08   Qualification

It shall be a condition of the Employee's employment that he is duly authorized to practise veterinary medicine in the Province of Ontario and is a member in good standing of the College of Veterinarians of Ontario.

2.00   TERM

2.01   Initial Term

The initial term of this Agreement shall be for a period of two (2) years from the date hereof (the "Term").

2.02   Automatic Renewal

Notwithstanding the Term as set out in Section 2.01 hereof, the Term of this Agreement shall be subject to automatic renewals for successive terms of one (1) year unless terminated by either party upon written notice of such termination delivered to the other party not less than sixty (60) days prior to the end of the then current Term.

3.00   COMPENSATION

3.01   Salary

The Employer agrees to pay to the Employee for the services provided by the Employee an annual salary in the amount of Forty Thousand

Dollars ($40,000.00) per annum payable in equal bi-weekly instalments of One Thousand, Five Hundred and Thirty-Eight Dollars and Forty-Six Cents ($1,538.46) subject to all statutory deductions including, but not limited to, income tax, Canada Pension Plan payments and Unemployment Insurance benefits.

3.02 Benefits

The Employee shall have the option of participating in the Employer's disability insurance plan at the Employee's own expense and shall be responsible for maintaining in full force a policy of Errors and Omissions Insurance as may be required by the Employer.

3.03 Salary Review

On each anniversary date of this Agreement, the Employer shall review the performance of the Employee with a view to increasing the annual salary set out in paragraph 3.01 and, in the event that the Employer determines that any increase is warranted in its sole discretion, then such increased salary shall be determined to be the salary paid to the Employee pursuant to the terms of this Agreement and the provisions of paragraph 3.01 shall apply mutatis mutandis to such increased salary.

4.00 PROPERTY OF EMPLOYER

4.01 Acknowledgement

The Employee hereby acknowledges that all documents related to the performance of his services as a veterinarian including, but not limited to, all contents of files, patient information and lists, accounting records, and all other file information (the "Materials"), shall be the sole property of the Employer and further agrees that the Materials shall be returned to the Employer upon twenty-four (24) hours' notice.

5.00 TERMINATION

5.01 Cause

The Employer may terminate this Agreement without notice or pay in lieu thereof for just cause including, but not limited to, the inability for any cause of the Employee to practise veterinary medicine or the Employee being suspended or membership privileges revoked from the College of Veterinarians of Ontario. In the event that this Agreement is so terminated, the Employer shall be entitled to withhold salaries due to the Employee and to set off same against damages, if any, incurred by the Employer as a result of the misconduct of the Employee.

5.02   Notice

The Employer may terminate this Agreement at any time without cause upon giving the Employee two (2) weeks' notice during the first year of this Agreement and one additional week for each subsequent year of employment by the Employee to a maximum of eight (8) weeks during the term of this Agreement or any renewal thereof.

5.03   Consequence of Termination

In the event that this Agreement or the employment of the Employee is terminated for any cause whatever, the following shall apply:

(a) All salaries which have been completely earned by the Employee and unpaid shall be paid to the Employee by the Employer subject to paragraph 5.01 hereof;

(b) All files, documents and records of the Employer in the possession of the Employee shall forthwith be delivered to the Employer; and

(c) If required by the Employer, the Employee shall make himself available to the Employer for a reasonable period after termination to provide any information relating to files in his possession at the date of termination.

6.00   GENERAL

6.01   Arbitration

All matters in difference in relation to this Agreement shall be referred to the arbitration of a single arbitrator. The parties shall agree upon and name an arbitrator in writing within fifteen (15) days after any party to this Agreement gives notice of arbitration to the other party, failing which an arbitrator shall be appointed or application of a party pursuant to the Arbitrators Act, RSO 1990. The award and determination of such arbitrator shall be binding upon the parties with respect to the matter so submitted and the costs thereof.

6.02   Notice

Any notice authorized or required by this Agreement to be given or served shall be in writing and deemed to be duly given or served if the same shall be delivered personally, or shall be sent by prepaid registered mail with return receipt requested to the following address:

(a)   In the case of the Employee:

R.R.# 10
Anywhere, Ontario   N1H 1Z1

(b)   In the case of the Employer:

123 Main Street
Anywhere, Ontario   N1H 9X9

In the event that notice shall be given by mail as aforesaid, it shall be conclusively deemed to have been given on the fourth (4th) business day after the date of mailing.

6.03   Assignment

The interest of the Employee under the Agreement shall not be assigned to any person without the consent in writing of the Employer. The Employer shall be entitled to assign its interest pursuant to this Agreement.

6.04   Governing law

This Agreement shall be governed by and construed in accordance with the laws of the Province of Ontario.

6.05   Severability

In the event that any Article or Section of this Agreement is held to be invalid or unenforceable by a court of competent jurisdiction, such invalidity or unenforceability shall not affect the remainder of the provisions hereof, but such parts shall be fully severable and this Agreement shall be construed and enforced as if such Article or Section had never been included herein.

6.06 <u>Entire Agreement</u>

This Agreement constitutes the entire agreement between the parties hereto and there are no representations or warranties or other terms except as herein contained in writing.

6.07 <u>Time of Essence</u>

Time shall in all respects be of the essence of this Agreement.

6.08 <u>Enurement</u>

This Agreement shall enure to the benefit of and be binding upon the parties hereto and their respective heirs, executors, administrators and assigns.

IN WITNESS WHEREOF the parties have duly executed this Agreement under seal.

**SIGNED, SEALED &
DELIVERED**
in the presence of

_____

Witness   Ima Newguy

_____

Witness   John White

_____

Witness   Jane Black

APPENDIX J

Employment Agreement (Lay)

FANTASY VETERINARY CLINIC
123 Main Street
Anyville, Ontario
L1L 8V9

(111) 123 - 4567

January 6, 1994

Ms. Jane White,
345 King Street,
Anyville, Ontario
L1L 2V8

Dear Jane:

Re.: Engagement as Veterinary Technician

Further to our office conference on December 28, 1993 we are pleased to provide you with this offer of employment with Fantasy Veterinary Clinic. We look forward to a long and mutually beneficial relationship with you on the following terms and conditions:

Position Title

You will be engaged by our practice as a veterinary techinician reporting to Dr. John White of our office to whom you shall have primary reporting responsibility. During the term of your engagement you shall be responsible for performing all of the usual functions of a veterinary technician including, but not limited to, assisting in veterinary surgery, performing routine therapeutic procedures under the direct supervision of the responsible veterinarian, patient records management, and post-operative observation.

Term

The term of your employment shall be for one (1) year commencing on January 10, 1994 and ending on January 9, 1995. The term of your engagement shall be subject to your satisfactorily completing a probationary period of three (3) months ending on March 9, 1994 at which time you may be offered a permanent position with our practice.

Your employment will be automatically renewed by us, provided that we do not give you written notice to the contrary at least twenty (20) days prior to the end of the initial term of your employment.

Remuneration

In exchange for your services we shall pay to you the sum of Thirty Thousand ($30,000.00) dollars per annum payable in equal bi-weekly payments of $1,153.84, subject to all usual statutory deductions for income tax, Canada Pension Plan and Unemployment Insuranance. Your salary shall be subject to annual review by the partners of the practice at least once each year after reviewing your performance with you.

Benefits

You are eligible, after your probationary period, to take part in our employees benefit program, including dental, short-term disability, long-term disability and group life insurance. Please advise our bookkeeper, Valerie Jones, if you would like to join these plans so that she can review the costs thereof with you.

In addition, you will be entitled to have veterinary services performed by our clinic at employee rates.

Expenses

You will be reimbursed for expenses incurred by you during the course of your employment, provided that they have been preapproved by a partner of the firm or upon ratification by the partners.

We shall pay you the sum of $0.31 per kilometer travelled on practice business for the use by you of your vehicle.

Termination

During the probationary period, your employment with us may be terminated at any time without notice. After the probationary period we shall provide with two weeks' notice of termination unless we have just cause for your termination, in which case we shall not be obliged to provide you with any notice. In the event that your engagement is renewed as provided for herein, we shall provide you with one additional week's notice of termination for every anniversary of your employment up to a maximum of eight weeks. At our option, we may provide you with a termination payment equal to the amount of salary you would have been entitled to for the period of notice then applicable.

Confidentiality

As you know, we are required to maintain the utmost confidentiality about client and patient matters; accordingly, any breach by you of this requirement will result in immediate termination without notice and without termination payment.

Acceptance

In the event that the terms of this correspondence are satisfactory to you, we would ask that you kindly acknowledge your acceptance of these terms in the area below and return the second copy of this letter to Dr. White.

Thank you for joining us. In the event that you require clarification with respect to these terms, please do not hesitate to contact me.

Yours very truly,

FANTASY VETERINARY CLINIC

per. John Black, DVM

<u>ACCEPTANCE</u>

The undersigned hereby acknowledges and accepts the terms of
this engagement letter.
Dated this 9th day of January, 1994.

_____

Jane White

236

APPENDIX K

Business Plan Checklist

Have you included?

☐ An introductory letter

☐ A title page

☐ A summary statement — brief description of your business

☐ Background information
 • Legal status of your firm
 • Start-up of your enterprise

☐ A description of the industry
 • Principal characteristics
 • Players
 • Trends
 • Barriers

☐ A description of your product or service
 • Assessment of strengths and weaknesses
 • Patents, trademarks, copyright protection
 • Technology you will be using

☐ A description of your management team
 • An organization chart
 • Curricula vitae
 • Management compensation

☐ Your marketing plan
 • Assessment of total market

- Assessment of target market
- Assessment of competition
- Assessment of your marketing advantage
- Your pricing policy
- Your selling policy
- Your distribution policy
- Your advertising/promotion plan
- Your services and warranties

☐ A description of the land, buildings, and equipment you will need
- Location
- Land requirements
- Equipment requirements

☐ A description of how you will operate
- Work flow
- Inventory control
- Supplies and material

☐ Personal references
- From banks
- From professionals
- From former employees

☐ A financial plan
- Your capital requirements
- Your sources of financing
- Cash flow budgets
- Projected income statements
- Pro forma balance sheet
- Break-even chart

☐ Risks and problems associated with your business and how to resolve them
- Worst-case scenario
- Avoidance of risk
- Impact of risk

APPENDIX L

Promissory Note

FORM 1407 (11-90)

_____ 19 ____

$ _____

ON DEMAND AFTER DATE, FOR VALUE RECEIVED _____ PROMISE TO

PAY TO _____ OR ORDER AT _____

THE ROYAL BANK OF CANADA _____ THE SUM OF

_____ DOLLARS

WITH INTEREST THEREON CALCULATED AND PAYABLE MONTHLY AT A RATE EQUAL TO THE ROYAL BANK OF CANADA'S PRIME INTEREST RATE PER ANNUM IN EFFECT FROM TIME TO TIME PLUS ___ % PER ANNUM AS WELL AFTER AS BEFORE MATURITY, DEFAULT AND JUDGMENT, WITH INTEREST ON OVERDUE INTEREST AT THE SAME RATE AS THE PRINCIPAL. AT THE DATE OF THIS NOTE SUCH PRIME INTEREST RATE IS ___ % PER ANNUM. THE UNDERSIGNED HEREBY WAIVE(S) PRESENTMENT FOR PAYMENT OF THIS PROMISSORY NOTE.

PRIME INTEREST RATE IS THE ANNUAL RATE OF INTEREST ANNOUNCED FROM TIME TO TIME BY THE ROYAL BANK OF CANADA AS A REFERENCE RATE THEN IN EFFECT FOR DETERMINING INTEREST RATES ON CANADIAN DOLLAR COMMERCIAL LOANS IN CANADA.

NAME			
LOAN ACCT. NO.	LOAN NO.		
CR. ACCT. NO.	TRANSIT NO.	CASUAL DISCOUNT ☐	MGR. INIT.
REN. $			

APPENDIX M

SECURITY AGREEMENT

FROM:

JOHN CLIENT
(hereinafter called the "Debtor)

TO:

DR. JOHN WHITE
(hereinafter called the "Secured Party")

1.0 <u>**OBLIGATIONS SECURED**</u>

1.1   The Debtor enters into this Security Agreement with the Secured Party for valuable consideration and as security for the repayment of all present and future indebtedness of the Debtor to the Secured Party hereinafter set forth, and all other indebtedness or sums of money payable by the Debtor to the Secured Party provided for in this Security Agreement (hereinafter collectively called the "Obligations"):

The Debt of the Debtor to the Secured Party for professional veterinary services as set out in a promissory note dated as of 1st day of October, 1994.

2.0 <u>**COLLATERAL**</u>

2.1   The following property and any and all additions, accessions and substitutions thereto and therefor and proceeds therefrom is for all purposes of this agreement deemed the Collateral:

1984 John Deere Tractor bearing serial number 12345678.

3.0 GRANT OF SECURITY INTEREST

3.1   The Debtor hereby mortgages and charges to the Secured Party as and by way of a fixed and specific mortgage and charge, and grants to the Secured Party a security interest in the Collateral.

3.2   If any portion of the Collateral is being acquired by the Debtor from the Secured Party, the Secured Party retains title to such Collateral.

3.3   The Debtor acknowledges that value has been given for the Security Agreement; and that the Debtor and the Secured Party intend each of the security interests in this Security Agreement to attach upon the execution of this Security Agreement.

3.4   The security herein is in addition to and not in substitution for any other security now or hereafter held by the Secured Party.

3.5   Until default, the Debtor may have possession of the Collateral.

4.0 DEBTOR'S COVENANTS

4.1 Warranty of Title

The Debtor covenants that it is, or to the extent that this Agreement states that the Collateral is to be acquired after execution hereof, will be, the owner of the Collateral free from any other lien, security interest or encumbrance, and that the Debtor will defend the Collateral against all claims and demands of all persons at any time claiming to Collateral or any interest therein.

4.2 Sale or Encumbrance of Collateral

The Debtor will not sell or offer to sell or otherwise transfer, or shall not lease, rent or otherwise part with possession of the Collateral, and will not create any liens upon, encumbrances in or security interests in the Collateral or any interest therein without the prior written consent of the third party.

4.3   Proceeds of Collateral

If any proceeds arising from any part of the Collateral shall be paid or become payable to the Debtor, the Debtor shall receive such proceeds as agent of the Secured Party and forthwith pay them over to the Secured Party.

4.4   Use and Protection of Collateral

(a) The Debtor shall:

    (i)   use the Collateral solely for the purpose for which it was manufactured or produced and intended in a proper and skilful manner;

    (ii) maintain the Collateral in good order and repair, and without material modification thereto unless the written consent of the Secured Party is first obtained;

    (iii) comply with all statutes or regulations in the ownership and use or operation of the Collateral;

    (iv) give the Secured Party any information as it may require at any time concerning the Collateral and the Debtor's affairs related thereto as the Secured Party may reasonably request, including location of the Collateral, repair and maintenance records, and shall provide the Secured Party with free and clear access to inspect the Collateral at any time on demand.

(b) Without limiting any other provision of this Security Agreement, the Debtor will take all steps and make all payments of money necessary to protect or preserve the Collateral that a prudent person would in like circumstances do, or as may be directed by the Secured Party from time to time.

(c) The Debtor shall forthwith advise the Secured Party in writing if the Collateral is lost, destroyed, stolen, or substantially altered or damaged in any way.

4.5   Insurance

(a) The Debtor will place insurance on the Collateral against risks of fire (including extended coverage) and theft, and such other risks as the

Secured Party may require, and in the case of motor vehicles, collision insurance with a deductible not exceeding Two Hundred and Fifty ($250.00) Dollars and comprehensive insurance with a deductible not exceeding Fifty ($50.00) Dollars. All such policies of insurance shall contain such terms and be in such form, for such periods and with such insurers as may be satisfactory to the Secured Party.

(b) The interest of the Secured Party shall be shown on all such insurance policies as mortgagee subject to a form of mortgage endorsed satisfactory to the Secured Party.

(c) The Debtor shall furnish the Secured Party with certificates or other evidence satisfactory to the Secured Party of such insurance. The Debtor shall duly and promptly pay all premiums and other sums payable for maintaining such insurance and provide the Secured Party with evidence satisfactory to the Secured Party thereof.

(d) Without imposing any obligation on the Secured Party, the Secured Party is hereby appointed as attorney for the Debtor in obtaining, adjusting, settling and cancelling such insurance.

4.6 Further Assurance

The Debtor shall at all times do, execute, acknowledge and deliver, or cause to be done, executed, acknowledged or delivered, all such further acts, deeds, transfers, assignments, security agreements and assurances as the Secured Party may reasonably require with respect to any matter provided for in this Security Agreement or related thereto.

4.7 Acts or Payments by Secured Party

Without imposing any obligations on the Secured Party, the Debtor hereby authorizes and appoints the Secured Party to perform all acts and make all agreements or payments required by the Debtor under this Agreement as its attorney or as its agent or on its own behalf as it shall in its discretion determine from time to time. The Debtor hereby indemnifies the Secured Party from and against all liabilities and claims arising therefrom, and shall forthwith pay to the Secured Party the amount of all such payments and any expenses incurred by the Secured Party acting under the provisions with this section.

5.0   EVENTS OF DEFAULT

5.1   The Debtor shall be in default under this Security Agreement upon the occurrence of any one of the following events:

(a)   The Debtor shall default under any of the Obligations;

(b)   The Debtor shall default in the due observance or performance of any covenant, undertaking or agreement heretofore or hereafter given to the Secured Party, whether contained herein or in any other document, or otherwise existing now or hereafter, and including any covenant or undertaking set out in any schedule to this Security Agreement;

(c)   An execution or any other process of any court shall become enforceable against the Debtor or a distress or analogous process shall be levied upon the property of the Debtor or any part thereof;

(d)   The Debtor shall become insolvent or commit an act of bankruptcy; or make an assignment in bankruptcy or a proposal in bankruptcy or a bulk sale of its assets; or a bankruptcy petition shall be filed or presented against the Debtor and not be bona fide opposed by the Debtor;

(e)   The Debtor shall cease to carry on business in the ordinary course;

(f)   Any other secured creditor of the Debtor shall take or threaten to take action or proceedings under any other security agreement or instrument creating a legal or equitable charge on the Collateral or any part thereof.

5.2   The Secured Party may waive any default herein referred to; provided always that no such waiver and no act or omission by the Secured Party under this Security Agreement shall in any manner whatsoever affect any subsequent default or the rights resulting therefrom.

6.0   REMEDIES ON DEFAULT

6.1   Upon any default under this Security Agreement the rights and remedies of the Secured Party set forth in this Section 6 may be exercised and the Secured Party may proceed to realize the security hereby constituted.

6.2   No remedy for the realization of the security hereof or for the enforcement of the rights of the Secured Party shall be exclusive of or dependent on any other such remedy, but any one or more of such remedies may from time to time be exercised independently or in combination.

6.3   The Secured Party may declare any or all of the Obligations to be immediately due and payable.

6.4   The Secured Party may enforce its rights by entry.

6.5   The Secured Party may enforce its rights by proceedings in any court of competent jurisdiction for the appointment of a receiver or receivers or for sale of the Collateral or any part thereof; or by any other action, suit, remedy or proceeding authorized or permitted hereby or by law or by equity.

6.6   The Secured Party may file such proofs of claim and other documents as may be necessary or advisable in order to have its claim lodged in any bankruptcy, winding-up or other judicial proceedings relative to the Debtor.

6.7   The Secured Party may take possession of, enter upon and lease or sell the whole or any part or parts of the Collateral. Any such sale may be made hereunder by public auction, by public tender or by private contract, with or without notice and with or without advertising. Such sale shall be on such terms and conditions as to credit or otherwise and as to upset or reserve bid or price as to the Secured Party in its sole discretion may seem advantageous and such sale may take place whether or not the Secured Party has taken possession of such property and assets.

6.8   Any and all payments made in respect of the Obligations from time to time and moneys realized from any securities held therefor (including moneys realized on any enforcement of this Security Agreement) may be applied to such part or parts of the Obligations as the Secured Party may see fit, and the Secured Party shall at all times and from time to time have the right to change any appropriation as the Secured Party may see fit.

7.0   **INTERPRETATION AND GOVERNING LAW**

7.1   This Security Agreement is entered into pursuant to and is governed by The Personal Property Security Act, R.S.O. 1990 (Ontario) insofar as the

Collateral (hereinafter defined) is located in Ontario, and except insofar as the Collateral is comprised of land.

7.2   In construing this Security Agreement:

(a)   Terms herein shall have the same meaning as defined in The Personal Property Security Act (Ontario) unless the context otherwise requires.

(b)   A reference to a person or the Debtor or any thing by number or gender shall be read and construed as demanded by the context, and, if more than one, shall apply and be binding upon each of them severally.

(c)   The terms "successors" shall include, without limiting its meaning, any corporation resulting from the amalgamation of a corporation with another corporation and, where the Debtor is a partnership, any new partnership resulting from the admission of new partners or any other change in the Debtor, including, without limiting the generality of the foregoing, the death of any or all of the partners.

8.0   <u>ADDITIONAL TERMS</u>

8.1   The Debtor agrees to pay all reasonable expenses, including solicitor's fees and disbursements, incurred by the Secured Party in the preparation, perfection and enforcement of this Security Agreement and the payment of such expense shall be secured hereby.

8.2   Nothing herein shall obligate the Secured Party to make any advance or loan or further advance or loan or to renew any note or extend any time for payment of any indebtedness or liability of the Debtor to the Secured Party.

8.3   This Security Agreement shall enure to the benefit of and be binding upon the respective heirs, executors, administrators, successors and assigns of the Debtor and the Secured Party.

8.4   The Debtor hereby acknowledges receipt of a copy of the within Security Agreement.

IN WITNESS WHEREOF this Security Agreement has been executed by the Debtor on the 1st day of October, 1994.

_____

John Client

APPENDIX N

Veterinary Invoice

Invoice   **Meadowlands Veterinary Hospital**

390 South Street, Fergus, Ontario N2K 3X6 Tel.   (519) 222-3434

Client's name

Client's address   Account   Invoice no.

Date		Cash	Cheque	MC/Visa	Charge	Init.
Name		Breed		Age	Sex	Colour
Doctor	Instructions/Dx					

1. Call		6. Health Services
Office		Deworm
Field		Dental
Emergency		Hospitalization
Recall		
2. Exam		
Routine		**7. Medical Treatment**
Reproductive		Injections
Prepurchase		
Health Certificate		
Ophthalmic		Medication
Radiology		
		Dressing
3. Vaccinations		
Tetanus/E & W/Flu		Fluid Therapy
Tetanus		
Flu		
Rhino		**8. Anaesthesia**
		Tranquillizer
		Local
4. Pharmacy		Nerve Block
		General
		9. Surgery
5. Lab		Castration
Fecal		Casticks
Coggins		Suture
		Surgery Room
GST		
PST		
Total Due		Total Balance

APPENDIX O

Sample Consent to Treatment Form

AUTHORIZATION TO PERFORM MEDICAL TREATMENT OR SURGERY

OWNER: .... ADDRESS: ....
CONTACT TELEPHONE #: .... ALTERNATE CONTACT #: ....
ANIMAL'S NAME: ....
SPECIES: .... BREED: .... COLOUR: .... SEX: ....

TO: ....
[Name of veterinary practice and veterinarian(s)]

PROCEDURE(S):

AUTHORIZATION:

1. I am the owner of the animal identified above. I am 18 years of age or older, and I have the authority to give this authorization and do so voluntarily, having been advised of all of the probable and material risks associated with this treatment.

2. Dr. .... has described the procedures identified above and has explained to my satisfaction the purpose for performing them and the risks involved with them. I realize that there can be no guarantee as to the animal's condition or the outcome of any procedures. In particular, I have been advised that, in the event that the treatment requires the use of anaesthesia, that there is a risk of death every time an anaesthetic is used and that I have been advised of the likelihood of such occurrence.

3. I authorize the performance of the identified procedures and the use of associated anaesthetics and other medications.

4. I also understand that unforeseen conditions may be revealed during the identified procedures which, in the opinion of the attending veterinarian, require more extensive or different procedures or treatments. I understand that reasonable efforts will be made to contact me to explain these procedures and treatments and obtain my instructions regarding them. However, if the efforts are unsuccessful, I authorize the performance of any procedures or treatments which are necessary in the professional opinion of the attending veterinarian.

5. I have agreed to pay $ .... for the above procedures and related clinic fees. I will pay this money at the time the animal is discharged and hereby acknowledge my indebtedness for this amount.

6. I have read and understand this authorization.

READ BEFORE SIGNING

DATE:

_____   _____
Witness   OWNER

APPENDIX P

Demand Letter

FANTASY VETERINARY HOSPITAL
123 Main Street
Anytown, Ontario
A1A 2B2

(111) 555-1212

August 23, 1994

Without Prejudice
Mr. Joe Client,
123 King Street,
Anytown, Ontario
A1A 2B3

Dear Mr. Client:

Re.: Outstanding Invoice Number 1234

A review of our accounting records indicates that the above-captioned invoice dated June 3, 1994 in the amount of $345.82 remains outstanding notwithstanding numerous reminder notices previously forwarded to you. To this end, we hereby demand payment of this outstanding invoice on or before August 30, 1993 failing which we propose to retain our legal counsel to commence proceedings to enforce payment of this debt, the costs of which will be borne by you.

Please make arrangements for the immediate payment of this overdue account so as to avoid further costs.

Yours very truly,
FANTASY VETERINARY HOSPITAL

per.   John White, DVM

JW/ab
cc. Legal Counsel

APPENDIX Q

Statement of Claim

Ontario Court (General Division)
Cour de l'Ontario (Division générale)

Ontario

.....ANYTOWN...... SMALL CLAIMS COURT
COUR DES PETITES CRÉANCES DE.......

CLAIM/CRÉANCE
Form/*Formule* 7A

Refer to No./*N° de référence*	1234	A.D. 19 **93**
Amount of Claim/*Montant de la créance*		$ **345.82**
Entry Fee/*Droits d'inscription*		$
Kilometers/*Kilométrage*		$
		$

If you wish to file a Claim, complete this form
Si vous désirez faire une demande, remplissez cette formule

WHEN REFERRING TO THIS DOCUMENT PLEASE USE NUMBER IN UPPER RIGHT CORNER
VEUILLEZ UTILISER LE NUMÉRO EN HAUT À DROITE COMME RÉFÉRENCE DE CE DOCUMENT

PLAINTIFF/*DEMANDEUR*

Name/*Nom*
JOHN WHITE, carrying on business as "FANTASY VETERINARY HOSPITAL"

DEFENDANT(S)/*DÉFENDEUR(S)*

Name/*Nom*
JOSEPH CLIENT

Street No./*N° et rue*	Address/*Adresse*	Apt. No./*N° d'app.*
123 King Street		

Borough/City/Ville/*Municipalité*	Postal Code/*Code postal*	Phone No./*N° de tél.*
Anytown, Ontario	A1A 2B3	(111) 222-3333

DEFENDANT/*DÉFENDEUR*

Name/*Nom*

Street No./*N° et rue*	Address/*Adresse*	Apt. No./*N° d'app.*

Borough/City/Ville/*Municipalité*	Postal Code/*Code Postal*	Phone No./*N° de tél.*

To the Defendant/*Au défendeur:*
The Plaintiff claims from you $ **345..82** .... and costs for the reason(s) set out below.
Le(s) demandeur(s) vous demand(ent) la somme de _____ $ plus les frais pour la(les) raison(s) indiquée(s) ci-après.

IF YOU DO NOT FILE A DEFENCE WITH THE COURT WITHIN TWENTY DAYS AFTER YOU HAVE RECEIVED THIS CLAIM, JUDGMENT MAY BE ENTERED AGAINST YOU.
SI VOUS NE DÉPOSEZ PAS DE DÉFENSE AUPRÈS DU TRIBUNAL DANS LES VINGT JOURS SUIVANT LA RÉCEPTION DE CETTE DEMANDE, UN JUGEMENT PEUT ÊTRE RENDU CONTRE VOUS.

TYPE OF CLAIM/*GENRE DE DEMANDE:*

☒ Unpaid account *Compte impayé* ☐ Contract *Contrat* ☐ Motor vehicle accident *Accident qui implique un véhicule automobile* ☐ Promissory note *Billet à ordre* ☐ Lease *Bail*

☐ Services rendered
Services rendus

☐ N.S.F. cheque
Chèque sans provision

☐ Damage to property
Dommages aux biens

☐ Other
Autres _____
(describe/préciser)

Reasons for Claim and Details/Raisons de la créance et détails:
(Explain what happened, where and when and the amounts of money involved)
(Indiquer les faits que donnent lieu à la demande, de même que le moment et l'endroit où ils se sont produits ainsi que les sommes d'argent en cause):

The Plaintiff is a professional veterinary practice conducting business in Anytown, Ontario and rendered such services to the Defendant on or about the 3rd day of June, 1993, at the request of the Defendant. On that date, the Plaintiff rendered its account for such services in the amount of $345.82 and despite numerous demands this account remains unpaid.

(Where claim is based on a document, attach a copy for each copy of the claim, or if it is lost or unavailable, explain why it is not attached.)
(Si la demande est fondée sur un écrit, annexer une copie de cet écrit pour chaque copie de la demande, ou si celui-ci a été perdu ou ne peut être produit, donner les motifs pour lesquels il n'est pas annexé.)

Make payments to the Court by certified cheque or money order./Faire les paiements à la Cour au moyen d'un chèque certifié ou d'un mandat.

Office use only/À l'usage du bureau

Plaintiff's Signature/Solicitor or
Agent's Name/Signature du demandeur   Mr. Legal Counsel
Nom de l'avocat ou du mandataire

Address/Adresse   133 Main Street

City/Borough/Ville/Municipalité   Anytown   Postal Code/Code postal A1A 2B4   Phone No./N° de tél (111) 222-3334

Date   September 1, 1993

CV 0330 (rev 03/90)

APPENDIX R

Veterinary Practice Valuation Method

The value of the practice shall be determined by the accountants for the practice who shall have the right to engage an independent veterinary practice valuator. The costs of such valuation shall be paid by the practice, and where the sale of an interest in the practice is effected subsequently from the same circumstances giving rise to the valuation, the transferor of the interest in the practice shall reimburse the practice for one-half (1/2) of the costs of such valuation.

In determining any value the valuator shall have regard to the following:

(a)   The effect of income tax on the practice shall be considered; and

(b)   the practice and assets shall be valued as a going concern.

APPENDIX S

Domestic Contract

THIS DOMESTIC CONTRACT made this 3rd day of February, 1994

B E T W E E N :

JOHN WHITE

- and -

JANE WHITE

1. **INTERPRETATION**

   1. In this contract:

      (a) "John" means the husband who is a party to this contract;

      (b) "Jane" means the wife who is a party to this contract;

      (c) "Act" means the Family Law Act as amended from time to time;

      (d) "property" or "net family property" has the meaning given by the Act;

      (e) "breakdown of the marriage" means:

         (i) the separation of the parties with no reasonable prospect that they will resume cohabitation;

        (ii)   the dissolution of their marriage; or

        (iii)   the annulment of their marriage;

(f)   "Practice" means the Fantasy Veterinary Hospital owned by John.

2.   BACKGROUND

1.   John is a Doctor of Veterinary Medicine carrying on practice in the City of Anyville, County of Anycounty;

2.   Jane is a chartered accountant carrying on practice in the City of Anyville, County of Anycounty;

3.   John and Jane intend to marry each other on 3rd day of June, 1994.

4.   John and Jane intend to live in the family residence, being a home located on lands and premises owned by John.

3.   PURPOSE OF CONTRACT

Each party intends by this contract:

(a)   to avoid any rights and obligations relating to property which arise or which may in the future arise at law or in equity from their marriage;

(b)   except as specifically provided by this contract, to elect and affirm that none of the property of either party will be divided between them except according to ownership; and

(c)   if there is a breakdown of the marriage, to make specific provision for the division after the breakdown of any increase in value of the Practice accruing between the effective date of this contract and the date of the breakdown of the marriage.

4.   AGREEMENT

Each party agrees with the other to be bound by the provisions of this contract.

5.   EFFECTIVE DATE OF CONTRACT

This contract takes effect on the date the parties marry.

6.   DOMESTIC CONTRACT

This is a marriage contract entered into under s. 52 of the Act and is a domestic contract which prevails over the same matters dealt with in the Act.

7.   FINANCIAL PROVISION

The responsibility for making financial provision for the family during cohabitation under the marriage will be assumed jointly by the parties in proportion to their respective financial abilities as may be agreed upon from time to time.

8.   SUPPORT AFTER BREAKDOWN OF MARRIAGE

If there is a breakdown of the marriage, each party will have such rights to receive financial support from the other and will be under such obligations to provide financial support to the other as are given or imposed upon each party by the Act.

9.   NO NET FAMILY PROPERTY

Under no circumstances will any property owned by either party or by them together, be included in the net family property of either party.

10.   WAIVER AND RELEASE

Each party:

(a)   waives all rights and entitlement, and

(b)   releases and discharges the other from all claims
that he or she has on the effective date of this contract or may later acquire under the Act or under the laws of any jurisdiction,

(c)   to a division of property or the value of property owned by the other,

(d)   to the equalization of their net family properties or other sharing of their net family property, and

(e)   to any property or value of property owned by the other,
on any basis notwithstanding the fact that

(f)   they are cohabiting,

(g)   they are married,

(h)   one party is improvidently depleting or may improvidently deplete his or her net family property,

(i)   they are separated,

(j)   a divorce is being or has been granted,

(k)   the marriage is being or has been declared a nullity, or

(l)   one party has died leaving the other surviving.

11.   DEEMED OWNERSHIP

Subject to an appropriate instrument in writing, the rule of law applying a presumption of resulting trust shall not be applied in questions of ownership of property between the parties, and

(a)   property transferred from one party to the other party shall be deemed to be owned by the party to whom the property is transferred;

(b)   property held in the name of one party shall be deemed to be owned by that party;

(c)   property held in the name of both parties as joint tenants shall be deemed to be owned by both parties as joint tenants; and

(d)   money on deposit in the name of both parties shall be deemed to be in the name of the parties as joint tenants.

12. NO OWNERSHIP UNLESS LEGAL OWNERSHIP

Except as provided by this contract, each party:

(a)   waives all rights and entitlement, and

(b)   releases and discharges the other from all claims

that he or she has on the effective date of this contract or may later acquire

(c)   in equity by way of constructive, implied or resulting trusts, or by way of any other doctrine in equity, and

(d)   at law under the Family Law Act and the laws of any jurisdiction,

to

(e)   compensation, and

(f)   any interest in property or the value of property owned by the other,

by reason of

(g)   the transfer of property to the other without any or any adequate payment or other consideration,

(h)   work, money or moneys worth contributed to the acquisition, management, maintenance, operation and improvement of property, or

(i)   any other fact or circumstance creating a beneficial interest in property.

13. RIGHT TO DEAL WITH SEPARATE PROPERTY

Each party may dispose of or encumber or otherwise deal with his or her property as he or she deems fit, free from any claim by the other as if he or she were unmarried.

14. FAMILY RESIDENCE

1.   Each party acknowledges that the family residence as defined herein is owned by John and each agrees with the other that it will remain the property of John.

2. If a breakdown of the marriage should occur, John will pay Jane a sum equal to one-half of any increase in the market value of the family residence accruing between the effective date of this agreement and the date of the breakdown of the marriage as determined under the next section of this agreement.

3. The sum will be payable within two years after the amount is determined.

4. Jane shall not be entitled to any lien and hereby covenants not to encumber any portion of the family residence.

15. **INCREASE IN MARKET VALUE**

1. The increase in market value of the family residence will be the increase occurring between:

    (a) the effective date of this contract, and

    (b) the date of the breakdown of the marriage.

2. The market value on the effective date of this contract is the total of $220,000.00.

3. The market value on the date of breakdown of the marriage will be the value determined by:

    (a) the agreement of the parties; or

    (b) the opinion of a single qualified appraiser selected by both parties; or

    (c) the agreement of a qualified appraiser selected by John and a qualified appraiser selected by Jane or if they cannot agree, then an average of the two appraisals completed. Appraisals shall be conducted as expeditiously as practicable.

16. **RIGHTS RELATING TO FAMILY RESIDENCE**

    Nothing in this contract restricts or modifies the rights of either party with respect to the possession of the family residence as owned by John, but each of the parties intends that if there should be a breakdown of the marriage, Jane will give John vacant possession of the family residence as of the date of the breakdown, although Jane is not and cannot be bound by this contract to do so.

17.   CONTENTS OF FAMILY RESIDENCE

If a breakdown of the marriage of the parties should occur, the contents of the family residence or any successor residence will be distributed between the parties according to ownership whether that ownership arises by way of purchase or gift, including gifts from the other party.

18.   NO PROPERTY TO BE A DIVISIBLE ASSET

No property owned by either party or by them jointly on the effective date of this contract or at any later time is or will be

   (a)   a family asset,

   (b)   family property, or

   (c)   property subject to division otherwise than according to ownership, under the Act or the law of any jurisdiction.

19.   RELEASE AGAINST BUSINESS INTERESTS

Without restricting the generality of the other waivers and releases given under this contract, except for any interest that is expressly granted by an instrument in writing or by this contract, John and Jane release one another from all claims that each may have on the effective date of this contract or may later acquire to all interests in any businesses in which either has an interest.

20.   RELEASE AGAINST THE ESTATE OF THE OTHER

Without restricting the other waivers and releases in this contract, and subject to transfers or bequests that either party may voluntarily make one to the other by way of a last will and testament, each party

   (a)   waives all rights, and

(b)   releases and discharges the other from all claims
that he or she has or may in the future acquire under the laws of any jurisdiction, particularly under the Act and the Succession Law Reform Act and their successors, entitling him or her upon the death of the other

     (c)   to a division of property owned by the other or to one-half the difference between their net family properties or to any other share of this difference, or to any share of the property of the other;

     (d)   if the other party dies leaving a will, to elect against taking under the Will in favour of receiving an entitlement equalizing their net family properties, or in favour of any other benefit;

     (e)   if the other party dies intestate, to elect to receive an entitlement in intestacy or to receive an entitlement equalizing their net family property;

     (f)   if the other party dies testate as to some property and intestate as to other property, to elect to take under the Will and to receive an entitlement in intestacy, or to receive an entitlement equalizing their net family properties;

     (g)   to share in the estate of the other under a distribution in intestacy in any manner whatsoever;

     (h)   to receive support as a dependant from the estate of the other in any manner whatsoever; and

     (i)   to act as executor and administrator of the estate of the other.

21.   **TRANSFER OR BEQUEST OF PROPERTY**
      TO OTHER PARTY

Either party may, by appropriate written instrument,

     (a)   convey or transfer during his or her lifetime, and

(b)   devise or bequeath for distribution after his or her death any property to the other, or appoint the other as executor of his or her estate. Nothing in this contract will limit or restrict in any way the right to receive any such conveyance, transfer, devise or bequest from the other, or, if so appointed, the right to act as executor or administrator of the estate of the other.

22.   **FINANCIAL DISCLOSURE**

Each party:

(a)   has fully and completely disclosed to the other the nature, extent and probable value of all his or her significant assets and all his or her significant debts or other liabilities existing at the date of this contract, and in addition to this disclosure,

(b)   has given all information and particulars about his or her assets and liabilities that have been requested by the other,

(c)   is satisfied with the information and particulars received from the other, and

(d)   acknowledges that there are no requests for further information or particulars that have not been met to his or her complete satisfaction.

23.   **AMENDMENT OF CONTRACT**

Any amendment of this contract will be unenforceable unless made in writing and signed by each party before a witness.

24.   **GOVERNING LAW**

This contract will be governed by the law of the Province of Ontario.

25.   **SEVERABILITY**

The invalidity or unenforceability of any provision of this contract will not affect the validity or enforceability of any other provision, and any invalid provision will be severable from this contract

26. CONTRACT TO SURVIVE DIVORCE

If a divorce is granted, or if the marriage is declared a nullity, the terms of this contract will survive the event and continue in force.

27. CONTRACT TO SURVIVE DEATH

This contract is intended to survive the death of a party or the parties and will be binding on the heirs, administrators, executors and assigns of the deceased party or parties.

28. INDEPENDENT LEGAL ADVICE

Each party acknowledges that he or she:

(a)   has had independent legal advice, or the opportunity to obtain independent legal advice;

(b)   understands his or her respective rights and obligations under this agreement; and

(c)   is signing this agreement voluntarily.

IN WITNESS WHEREOF Jane has hereunto set her hand and seal this 3rd day of June, 1994.

IN WITNESS WHEREOF John has hereunto set his hand and seal this 3rd day of June, 1994.

SIGNED, SEALED
AND DELIVERED

in the presence of

_____

As to the execution by John White

Witness's Name:

Address:

Occupation:

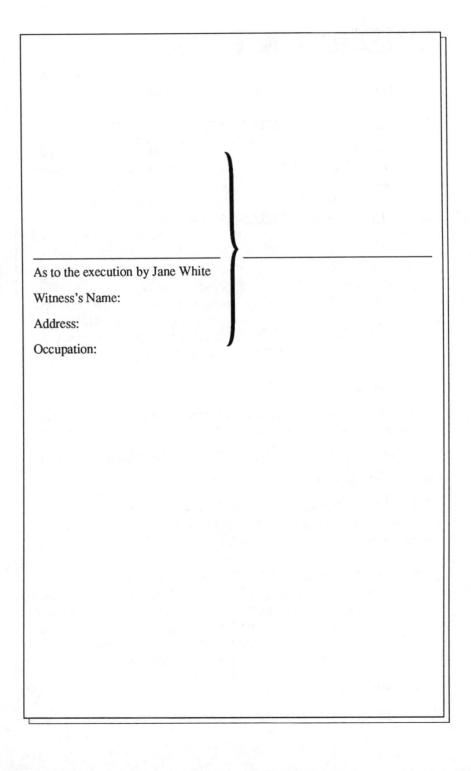

As to the execution by Jane White

Witness's Name:

Address:

Occupation:

APPENDIX T

Will Clauses Concerning Animals

Sample Bequest for Maintenance of Pet

To set aside the sum of $5,000.00 and to keep the said sum invested and to use the income and capital or so much thereof as my Trustees consider advisable for the maintenance and welfare of my dog and trusted friend, Fido and to assure that he is properly fed and given proper care for the period of twenty (20) years from my death, if my dog shall so long live. Any income not so used in any years to be added to the capital of the sum and dealt with as part thereof, and upon the death of my dog, Fido, whereupon the expiration of the said period, whichever event shall occur first, the said sum together with any accumulation of income shall form part of the residue of my estate.

Bequest of Pet

To transfer and deliver to my friend, JOHN WHITE, my two cats, Fifi and Tipper, together with all the equipment used in connection with them and owned by me at the time of my death.

Gift to Individual for Care of Pet

I give to my friend, JOHN WHITE, the sum of $2,000.00 for the purpose of enabling him to carry out the trust with respect to my cats which I have already communicated to him in my lifetime. For greater certainty I set out my intentions in writing such that it is my wish that after my death the said JOHN WHITE shall find a good home for my cats and that they shall be kept together. The home so selected should be one with proper facilities so that the cats can lead a happy and healthy life, and should be one where they will have kind human companionship to which they are accustomed. The sum set out herein can be used by the said JOHN WHITE in his sole discretion to make the desired arrangements.

APPENDIX U

Veterinarian's Oath

Being admitted to the profession of Veterinary Medicine, I solemnly dedicate myself and the knowledge I possess to the benefit of society, to the conservation of our livestock resources and to the relief of suffering animals. I will practice my profession conscientiously with dignity. The health of my patients, the best interest of their owners, and the welfare of my fellow man will be my primary considerations. I will at all times be humane and temper pain with anaesthesia where indicated. I will not use my knowledge contrary to the laws of humanity or in contravention of the ethical code of my profession. I will uphold and strive to advance the honour and noble traditions of the Veterinary Profession. These pledges I make freely in the eyes of God and upon my honour.

INDEX